RELIABILITY ASSURANCE FOR MEDICAL DEVICES, EQUIPMENT AND SOFTWARE

Richard C. Fries, PE, CRE

Printing History:
Reliability Assurance for Medical Devices, Equipment and Software

First Edition, ISBN: 0-935184-20-1

© Copyright, 1991 by Interpharm Press, Inc.
1358 Busch Parkway
Buffalo Grove, IL 60089, USA

Telephone: 708/459-8480
Telefax: 708/459-6644

To
June
who gives so much, asks so little
and makes life worth living
and
to
Tom and **Matt**
young men who make me proud to be their Dad

Contents

                                                                    Page
Preface xiii
Acknowledgements xvi

The Basics of Reliability

1. The Science of Reliability

1.1	History of Reliability	2
1.2	Reliability vs Unreliability	2
1.3	Reliability vs Quality	3
1.4	The Definition of Reliability	4
1.5	Reliability Assurance	5
1.6	Types of Reliability	6
1.6.1	Electronic Reliability	6
1.6.1.1	Infant Mortality	7
1.6.1.2	Useful Life	7
1.6.1.3	Wearout	7
1.6.2	Mechanical Reliability	8
1.6.3	Software Reliability	9
1.7	Device Reliability.	9
1.8	Optimizing Device Reliability	10
1.9	Reliability's Effect on Medical Devices	11
1.10	Summary	11
1.11	References	11

2. Reliability and the Concept of Failure

2.1	Closely Related Terms	13
2.2	Failure	15
2.3	Time Related Failures	15

2.3.1   Early Failures 15
2.3.2   Chance Failures 16
2.3.3   Wearout Failures 16
2.4   Operational Failures 16
2.4.1   Catastrophic Failure 16
2.4.2   Drift Failure 17
2.4.3   Degradation Failure 17
2.4.4   Intermittent Failure 17
2.5   Reliability Parameters 19
2.5.1   Failure Rate 19
2.5.2   Mean Time Between Failure 20
2.5.3   Reliability 20
2.6   Failure Correction 21
2.7   Summary 21
2.8   References 21

3. Reliability, Standards and Regulations

3.1   Food and Drug Administration (FDA) 23
3.2   Basic Standards Organizations 27
3.2.1   Underwriters Laboratory 28
3.2.2   International Electrotechnical Commission 28
3.2.3   Canadian Standards Association 29
3.2.4   National Fire Protection Association 29
3.3   Other Standards Organizations 30
3.3.1   Association for Advancement of
             Medical Instrumentation 30
3.3.2   British Standards Institute 30
3.3.3   International Special Committee on
             Radio Interference 31
3.3.4   Department of Health 31
3.3.5   European Committee for Standardization 31
3.3.6   European Committee for Electrotechnical
             Standardization 32
3.3.7   Institute of Electrical and Electronic Engineers ... 32
3.3.8   International Organization for Standardization 32
3.3.9   Japanese Standards Association 33
3.4   Contacting the Organizations 33
3.5   European Harmonization 33
3.5.1   Regulatory Institutions 35
3.5.1.1   The Commission 35
3.5.1.2   The Council 35

3.5.1.3	The European Parliament	36
3.5.1.4	The European Court of Justice	36
3.5.2	Regulatory Schemes	36
3.5.3	Medical Device Classification	38
3.5.4	European Free Trade Area	38
3.6	Summary	38
3.7	References	39

The Product Development Process

4. Overview of the Product Development Process

4.1	Feasibility	43
4.2	Design	43
4.3	Validation	44
4.4	Manufacturing	45
4.5	Field Operation	46
4.6	Feedback	46
4.7	Summary	47
4.8	References	47

5. The Feasibility Phase

5.1	Customer Survey	49
5.2	Product Specification	50
5.3	Reliability Goal	51
5.4	Specification Review	53
5.5	Summary	53
5.6	References	54

6. The Design Phase –The Device

6.1	System Specification	55
6.1.1	Hardware/Software Compatibility	55
6.2	Design Review	56
6.3	Reliability Plan	56
6.4	Reliability Report	57
6.5	Summary	58
6.6	References	58

7. The Design Phase –Hardware

7.1	Safety	59
7.2	Block Diagram	61
7.3	Redundancy	61
7.3.1	Active Redundancy	61

7.3.2   Standby Redundancy..............................63
7.4   Component Selection.............................64
7.4.1   Component Fitness for Use......................64
7.4.2   Component Criticality..........................65
7.4.3   Component Reliability..........................67
7.4.4   Component History 69
7.4.5   Component Safety 69
7.5   Component Classification 70
7.6   Component Derating 71
7.7   Safety Margin 72
7.8   Load Protection 73
7.9   Environmental Protection.......................74
7.10   Product Misuse 74
7.11   Initial Reliability Prediction 75
7.11.1   Parts Count Prediction 76
7.11.2   Parts Count Prediction Example 77
7.12   Design Reviews 86
7.13   Summary 90
7.14   References.....................................90

8. The Design Phase – Software

8.1   Hardware vs Software 93
8.2   Software Reliability...........................93
8.3   Software and the FDA...........................96
8.4   Software Quality Assurance 98
8.4.1   Software Specification 99
8.4.2   Structured Design 99
8.4.3   Module Interaction 100
8.4.4   Software Reviews..............................101
8.5   Software Safety 103
8.6   Software Metrics 104
8.6.1   Mc Cabe's Complexity 105
8.6.2   Halstead Measures 106
8.6.2.1   Vocabulary of the Software....................106
8.6.2.2   Length of the Program 106
8.6.2.3   Volume of Software 107
8.6.3   Other Metrics.................................107
8.6.4   Computer Aided Metrics........................107
8.7   Software Failures.............................108
8.8   Coding..109
8.9   Summary 109
8.10   References....................................109

9. The Validation Phase – Hardware

9.1	The Test	113
9.2	Test Protocol	114
9.2.1	Type of Test	114
9.2.1.1	Long Term Reliability Testing	114
9.2.1.2	Event Testing	115
9.2.1.3	Overstress Testing	115
9.2.1.4	Environmental Testing	115
9.2.1.5	Other Types of Testing	115
9.2.1.5.1	Time Related	115
9.2.1.5.2	Failure Related	115
9.2.2	Purpose of the Test	116
9.2.3	Failure Definition	116
9.2.4	Determining Sample Size and Test Length	116
9.2.5	Sample Test Protocol	119
9.3	Standard Tests	121
9.3.1	Cycle Testing	121
9.3.2	Typical Use Testing	121
9.3.3	10 x 10 Testing	121
9.3.4	Fault Tree Analysis	122
9.3.4.1	The Fault Tree Process	123
9.3.5	Failure Modes and Effects Analysis	128
9.4	Accelerated Testing	131
9.4.1	Increasing Sample Size	131
9.4.2	Increasing Test Severity	131
9.4.3	Sudden Death Testing	133
9.4.3.1	Weibull Analysis	134
9.4.3.2	Confidence Limits	135
9.4.3.3	The Shape of Weibull Plots	138
9.4.3.4	The Sudden Death Test	138
9.5	Summary	144
9.6	References	146

10. The Validation Phase – Software

10.1	Software Testing	147
10.2	Test Principles	148
10.3	Verification and Validation Plan	148
10.3.1	Test Strategies	149
10.3.1.1	Black Box Testing	149
10.3.1.2	White Box Testing	149
10.3.2	Test Completion Criteria	149
10.3.3	Failure Definition	150

10.3.3.1   Hard Failure 150
10.3.3.2   Soft Failure 150
10.4   Verification and Validation Activity 150
10.4.1   Failure Mode Analysis 151
10.4.2   Structured Software Testing 151
10.4.2.1   Component Testing 151
10.4.2.2   Integration Testing 151
10.4.2.3   System Testing 151
10.4.2.4   Acceptance Testing 152
10.4.3   Test Data for Reliability Calculations 152
10.5   Verification and Validation Report 152
10.6   Validation Software Review 153
10.7   Summary 153
10.8   References 153

11. The Validation Phase – The Device

11.1   Hardware/Software Compatibility 155
11.2   Environmental Testing 156
11.2.1   Operating Temperature Testing 156
11.2.2   Storage Temperature Testing 157
11.2.3   Thermal Shock Testing 157
11.2.4   IIumidity Testing 157
11.2.5   Mechanical Shock Testing 159
11.2.6   Mechanical Vibration Testing 159
11.2.7   Impact Testing 160
11.2.8   Electrostatic Discharge 161
11.2.9   Electromagnetic Compatibility 161
11.3   Safety Analysis 162
11.4   Beta Evaluation 163
11.5   Reliability Demonstration 165
11.6   Summary 166
11.7   References 166

12. The Validation Phase – Data Analysis

12.1   Failure Rate 169
12.2   Mean Time Between Failures 170
12.2.1   Time Terminated, Failed Parts Replaced 171
12.2.2   Time Terminated, No Replacement 172
12.2.3   Failure Terminated, Failed Parts Replaced 172
12.2.4   Failure Terminated, No Replacement 173
12.2.5   No Failures Observed 174
12.3   Reliability 175

12.4	Confidence Level	176
12.5	Confidence Limits	177
12.5.1	Time Terminated Confidence Limits	177
12.5.2	Failure Terminated Confidence Limits	178
12.6	Minimum Life	179
12.7	Graphical Analysis	179
12.7.1	Pareto Analysis	179
12.7.2	Graphical Plotting	181
12.7.3	Weibull Plotting	182
12.8	Summary	185
12.9	References	185

Manufacturing and Field Use of Devices

13. The Manufacturing Phase

13.1	Product Release	187
13.1.1	Conditional Release	189
13.1.2	Final Release	189
13.2	Structured Manufacturing Process	189
13.2.1	Design Involvement	189
13.2.2	Component Activity	190
13.2.2.1	Incoming Requirements	190
13.2.2.2	Component Qualification	191
13.2.2.3	Lot Control	191
13.2.3	Burn-In Activity	191
13.2.3.1	To Burn-In or not to Burn-In	192
13.2.3.2	Length of Burn-In	192
13.2.3.3	Types of Burn-In	192
13.2.4	Assembly	193
13.2.5	Test and Inspection	193
13.2.6	System Burn-In	194
13.2.7	Failure Analysis	195
13.2.8	Statistical Process Control	195
13.2.9	Electrostatic Discharge Protection	195
13.3	The FDA and Good Manufacturing Practices	196
13.3.1	Written Procedures	197
13.3.2	Application of the GMP	197
13.3.3	Quality Assurance Requirements	198
13.3.4	GMP Inspections	198
13.3.4.1	Details of the Inspection	199
13.3.5	Sanctions	200
13.4	Summary	200
13.5	References	201

14. The Field Operation Phase

14.1   Analysis of Field Service Reports 203
14.1.1   The Database 204
14.1.2   Data Analysis...............................205
14.2   Failure Analysis of Field Units 211
14.3   Warranty Analysis...........................213
14.4   The GMP and Field Data 213
14.4.1   Complaint Handling 213
14.4.2   Medical Device Reporting 214
14.4.3   Failure Investigation 215
14.4.4   Trending 215
14.4.5   Product Recalls 215
14.5   Summary 216
14.6   References.................................216

15. The Feedback Phase

15.1   Engineering 220
15.2   Manufacturing Engineering 220
15.3   Regulatory Affairs..........................220
15.4   Reliability Assurance 220
15.5   Quality Assurance 221
15.6   Marketing..................................221
15.7   Legal 221
15.8   Top Management 221
15.9   Summary 221

Appendix 1 Chi Square Table 223
Appendix 2 Percent Rank Tables 225
Appendix 3 Standards and Regulatory
           Organization Addresses 241
Appendix 4 Reliability Glossary 245
Index 257

Preface

Reliability Assurance provides the theoretical and practical tools whereby the probability and capability of systems and their components to perform required functions can be specified, predicted, designed-in, tested and demonstrated. Reliability Assurance is an integral part of the product development process and of problem solving activities related to manufacturing and field failures. Analysis of component and device failures provides a valuable source of information for product development personnel.

Reliability is more than a science; it is also a philosophy, a way of thinking about how professional activities are conducted. It involves structuring those activities so they are planned before action is taken and problems are foreseen so they may be eliminated before they occur. The philosophy behind reliability may be found in the question heard many times within product development teams:

> Why is there never enough time to do it right,
> but always enough time to do it over?

The name of the game is doing things right the first time. The benefits in time and money saved are worth the effort.

This book provides a practical approach to the formation and operation of a Reliability Assurance program. The emphasis of the book is on the practical, "hands-on" approach. The mathematics included in the text is that necessary to conduct everyday tasks; equations, where needed, are merely given, not derived. It is assumed the reader has a basic knowledge of statistics. For those wishing to delve deeper into the mathematics of the subject, references are given at the end of each chapter.

The book is divided into three sections, simulating a typical approach to Reliability Assurance. First, the basics of reliability must be mastered.

Second, the knowledge is applied in the design and development of a medical device. Third, the knowledge is applied in the manufacturing of the device and in the monitoring of the device in the field.

The first section, "The Basics of Reliability," is a review of the material necessary to an understanding of reliability. It begins with a review of the history of reliability. This leads to a formal definition of reliability and its relation to quality. The various types of reliability are discussed, including optimizing device reliability.

The concept of failure is an integral part of reliability. This concept is discussed and a formal definition given. The failure concept is then related to various reliability parameters such as Mean Time Between Failure.

Section one concludes with a review of pertinent domestic and international standards and their relation to the production of a safe, effective and reliable medical device. Regulatory agencies for medical devices are also discussed.

Section two, "The Product Development Process," looks first at an overview of the various phases of the process and then at each phase in detail. The Design Phase and Validation Phase are each divided into three areas: hardware, software and device. Hardware and software are discussed in separate chapters. The device chapter discusses how the hardware and software come together and interact. Current guidelines from the Food and Drug Administration and other regulatory agencies are reviewed.

Section three, "Manufacturing and Field Use of Devices," looks at the manufacturing process and field use of devices not as separate entities, but as a continuation of the Product Developoment Process. A device may be designed reliably, but if it is not manufactured and serviced reliably, it will not be a success.

The chapter on the manufacturing process discusses the current Good Manufacturing Practices regulation and how it relates to manufacturing activities. A review of typical FDA inspection criteria is also discussed to better prepare for an inspection.

The chapter on field use discusses the establishment of a database for monitoring field activity. This fits well with the FDA requirement for trending of field data. The section closes with a discussion of feedback of field information to appropriate Product Development personnel, where it may lead to device changes or enhancements.

Mathematical tables, addresses for standards/regulatory organizations and a glossary are included in the appendices. The glossary contains definitions of terms used throughout the text.

Reliability Assurance is essential to the success of any medical device company. It helps develop a more profitable product, contributes to a more satisfied customer base, reduces the risk of liability and builds confidence in meeting the requirements of standards and regulatory organizations. It is hoped this text will assist in establishing and operating a viable Reliability Assurance program.

Acknowledgments

I am deeply indebted to many people for their encouragement, help and constructive criticism in making this book possible.

I especially want to thank my family, June, Tom and Matt, who constantly encouraged me and who sacrificed much in the way of time together and activities in allowing me to put this book together. This book is as much theirs as it is mine.

I want to thank Helen Grenier whose lifelong committment to education has been a constant inspiration.

I want to thank Dr. George H. Grenier who gave me my first slide rule and introduced me to the world of engineering.

I want to thank Dr. Dimitri Kececioglu, at the University of Arizona, who first introduced me to the philosophy of Reliability and made it more than a science, but a way of conducting one's professional activities.

Special thanks to Peg Rickard and Ray Riddle who reviewed the draft and provided new insights on the material. Ray also provided valuable assistance in reviewing the technical material and providing guidance on the standards and regulations.

1

The Science of Reliability

The design and functional complexity of medical devices have expanded during the past 50 years. Devices have progressed from the use of a metronome circuit for the initial cardiac packemaker to functions that include medical bookkeeping, electrocardiogram analysis, anesthesia delivery, laser surgery, magnetic resonance imaging (MRI) and intravenous delivery systems which adjust dosages based upon patient feedback. With software controlling functionality in the majority of medical devices, the opportunities for more complex capabilities are virtually limitless.

As functionality becomes more intricate, certain concerns arise from both the user and the patient population. Imagine yourself a patient having an exam using a medical device, such as a MRI device. Prior to and during the exam, you are concerned about three things: You want the device to function without causing you injury. You want the device to do what it is supposed to do, so the test results are accurate and meaningful. You want the device to work for a long time - at least until your exam is completed. The user has the same three concerns, although the desire to have the device operate for a longer time than one exam session is more acute. Thus both user and patient want the device to be safe, effective and reliable. This is what the FDA wants as well.

In 1976, the Medical Device Amendments to the Federal Food, Drug and Cosmetic Act gave the Food and Drug Administration (FDA) the authority to regulate medical devices during most phases of development. Since that time, the FDA has required, in all its regulations, that all medical devices be safe and effective for their intended use. In the mid-'80s, the FDA added the term reliability to this requirement. To understand why, we need to examine what reliability is and how it affects medical devices.

1

1.1 History of Reliability

Reliability as a science originated during World War II, when the Germans first introduced the concept to improve the operation of their V-1 and V-2 rockets. Prior to this time, most equipment was essentially mechanical and failures could usually be isolated to a simple part. Products were expected to be reliable and safety margins in stress-strength, wear or fatigue conditions were employed to assure it. As electronics began to grow, so did reliability.

From 1945 to 1950, various military studies were conducted in the United States on equipment repair, maintenance costs and failure of electronic equipment. As a result of these studies, the Department of Defense established an ad hoc committee on reliability in 1950. In 1952, this committee became a permanent group, known as the Advisory Group on the Reliability of Electronic Equipment (AGREE). In 1957, this group published a report that led directly to a specification on the reliability of military electronic equipment.

In the early sixties, the field of reliability experienced growth and widespread application in the aerospace industry, especially following the failure of Vanguard TV3 and several satellites. During this time engineers began to realize that to improve reliability, one must eliminate the source of failures. This led to the first Physics of Failure Symposium in 1962. This was followed by a period of growth in other highly technical areas, such as computers.

Today many industries and government agencies employ specialists in the area of reliability. Reliability is moving in the direction of more realistic recognition of causes and effects of failures, from the system to the component level. These companies have come to realize that poor reliability is costly, leads to a poor reputation and the subsequent loss of market share. Industries that are regulated must comply with reliability requirements established by the regulating agencies.

1.2 Reliability vs Unreliability

Reliability, a term that has been used extensively, is greatly misunderstood. Reliability has been described by some as a group of statisticians spewing endless streams of data. Others have described it as testing a device "ad nauseum", in order to make it reliable. Reliability is neither of these.

Reliability is a characteristic that describes how good a device really is. It is a measure of the dependability of the device. It is a characteristic that must be planned for, designed and manufactured into a device.

The inclusion of reliability in manufacturing is important, because no matter how reliably a device is designed, it will not be a success unless it is manufactured and serviced reliably. Reliability is a philosophy that dictates how good a device will be.

Unreliability is a measure of the potential for failure of a device. It is the result of the lack of planning for design and manufacturing activities. It is a philosophy that states the manufacturer does not care about how good their device will be. The consequences of such a philosophy include:

> High cost
> Wasted time
> Customer inconvenience
> Poor reputation.

Because reliability is preferable to unreliability, processes should be instituted to avoid the causes of unreliability, including:

> Improper design
> Use of inappropriate materials
> Manufacturing errors
> Assembly and Inspection errors
> Improper testing
> Improper packaging and shipping
> Improper startup
> User abuse
> Misapplication.

1.3 Reliability vs Quality

The term "quality" may be defined as:

> The degree of conformance to specification and/or workmanship standards.

Quality refers to this conformance at a particular instant of time. Thus, we may speak of the quality of a component at incoming, the quality of an assembly in Manufacturing test, or the quality of a device at a pre-operation checkout.

The traditional concept of quality does not include the notion of a timebase. A medical device is assessed against a specification or set of attributes. Having passed the assessment, the device is delivered to a customer, accompanied by a warranty, so that the customer is relieved of the cost implications of early failures. The customer, upon accepting the device, realizes that it might fail at some future time, hopefully far into the future. This approach provides no measure of the quality of the device outside the warranty period. It assumes this is the customer's responsibility and not the company's.

The need for a time-based measure of quality is satisfied by reliability and marks the difference between the traditional concept of quality and the modern approach to reliability. Reliability is described as the science of estimating, controlling and managing the probability of failure over time, such as the five year expected life of a device or an eight hour operation.

The modern concept of reliability concerns itself with quality over time. If the medical device is not only assessed against a specification or set of attributes, but is additionally designed for a Mean Time Between Failures of 5 years prior to being sent to the customer, reliability is being designed into the product. A company must realize that, if they want to be successful and build a satisfied customer base, the responsibility for the quality of the device outside the warranty period belongs to them.

1.4 The Definition of Reliability

This idea of quality over a period of time is reflected in the more formal definition of reliability:

> The probability, at a desired confidence level, that a device will perform a required function, without failure, under stated conditions, for a specified period of time.

This definition contains four key requirements:

> To *perform a required function*, the function must have been specified through such activities as customer and/or market surveys. Thus, reliability requires the device to be fully specified prior to design.

> To *perform without failure*, the normal operation of the device must be defined, in order to establish what a failure is. This activity also includes anticipating the misuse to which the device could be subjected and designing around it.

> To *perform under stated conditions*, the environment in which the device will operate must be specified. This includes typical temperature and humidity ranges, methods of shipping, shock and vibration experienced in normal usage and interference from associated equipment or to other equipment.

To *operate for a specified period of time*, the life expectancy of the device must be defined as well as the typical daily usage.

In summary, reliability assumes that preliminary thought processes have been completed and that the device and its environment have been thoroughly defined. These conditions make the task of the designer easier and less costly in time and effort. It assumes that failure-free or failure-tolerant design principles are used. It assumes manufacturing processes are designed so that they will not reduce the reliability of the device.

1.5 Reliability Assurance

Reliability Assurance is the science that provides the theoretical and practical tools whereby the functionality of a component or device may be evaluated with a certain confidence. Reliability Assurance includes:

Establishing reliability in design by use of failure-free or failure-tolerant principles

Verifying reliability by well-designed test procedures

Producing reliability by proper manufacturing processes

Assuring reliability by good quality control and inspection

Maintaining reliability by proper packaging and shipping practices

Assuring operational reliability by proper field service and appropriate operations and maintenance manuals

Improving reliability throughout the life of the device by information feedback on field problems and a system to address these issues.

The functions of Reliability Assurance form a structured approach to the life cycle of a medical device. They are discussed in detail in subsequent chapters.

Reliability Assurance, like any science, depends upon other technical areas as a base for its functionality. These include:

Basic mathematics and statistics
Current regulatory standards
Design principles
Software Quality Assurance

System interface principles
Human factors
Cost/benefit analysis
Common sense.

1.6 Types of Reliability

Reliability is composed of three primary subdivisions, each with their own particular attributes:

Electronic reliability
Mechanical reliability
Software reliability.

1.6.1 Electronic Reliablity

Electronic reliability (Figure 1.1) is a function of the age of a component or assembly. The failure rate is defined in terms of the number of malfunctions occurring during a period of time. The graph of electronic reliability is divided into three distinct time periods:

Infant mortality
Useful life
Wearout.

Figure 1.1 Electronic Life Curve

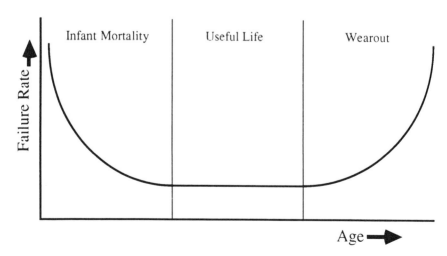

1.6.1.1 Infant Mortality

Infant mortality is the beginning of the life of an electronic component or assembly. This period is characterized by an initial high failure rate, which decreases rapidly and then stabilizes. These failures are caused by gross, built-in flaws due to faulty workmanship, bad processes, manufacturing deviations from the design intent or transportation damage. Examples of early failures include:

> Poor welds or seals
> Poor solder joints
> Contamination on surfaces or in materials
> Voids, cracks, or thin spots on insulation
>   or protective coatings.

Many of these failures can be prevented by improving the control over the manufacturing process, by screening components or by burn-in procedures. Improvements in design or materials are necessary for these manufacturing deviations.

1.6.1.2 Useful Life

The useful life period of a component or assembly, the largest segment of the life cycle, is characterized by a constant failure rate. During this period, the failure rate reaches its lowest level and remains relatively constant. Failures are either stress-related or occur by chance and are the most difficult to repeat or analyze.

1.6.1.3 Wearout

The final period in the life cycle occurs when the failure rate begins to increase rapidly. Wearout failures are due primarily to deterioration of the design strength of the components or assemblies, as a consequence of operation or exposure to environmental fluctuations. Such deterioration may result from:

> Corrosion or oxidation
> Insulation breakdown or leakage
> Ionic migration of metals on surfaces or in vacuum
> Frictional wear or fatigue
> Shrinkage and cracking in plastics.

A preventive maintenance program in which components are replaced prior to reaching the wearout period can prevent wearout failures.

1.6.2 Mechanical Reliability

Mechanical reliability (Figure 1.2) differs from electronic reliability in its reaction to the aging of a component or assembly. Mechanical components or assemblies begin their life cycle at a failure rate of zero and experience a rapidly increasing failure rate. This curve approximates the wearout portion of the electronics life curve.

Figure 1.2 Mechanical Life Curve

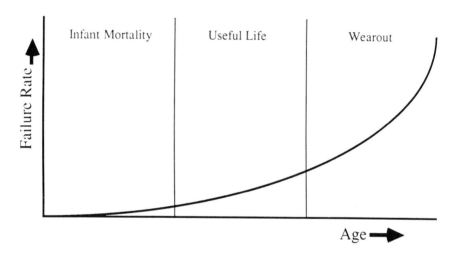

Mechanical failures are due primarily to deterioration of the design strength of the component or assembly. Such deterioration may result from:

> Frictional wear
> Shrinkage and/or cracking in plastics
> Fatigue
> Surface erosion
> Corrosion
> Creep
> Material strength deterioration.

Optimization of mechanical reliability occurs with timely elimination of components or assemblies through preventive maintenance, before the failure rate raches unacceptably high levels.

1.6.3 Software Reliability

Software is not subject to the physical constraints of electronic and mechanical components. Software reliability consists of the process of preventing failures through structured design and detecting and removing errors in the coding. Once all bugs are removed, the program will operate without failure forever (Figure 1.3).

Software failures are due primarily to:

> Specification errors
> Design errors
> Typographical errors
> Omission of symbols.

These are discussed in detail in Chapter 8.

Figure 1.3 Software Life Curve

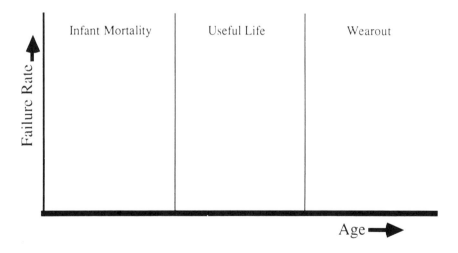

1.7 Device Reliability

The life cycle of any medical device may be represented by the Reliability Bathtub Curve (Figure 1.4). It is a graph of failure rate versus the age of the device.

Figure 1.4 Reliability Bathtub Curve

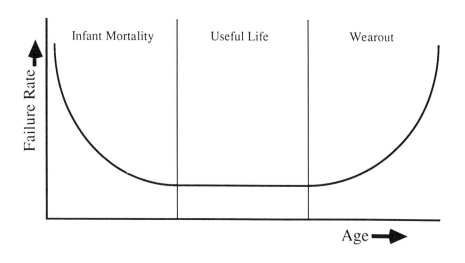

The graph is identical to that for electronics described above. As with the electronics life curve, there are three distinct time periods:

Infant mortality
Useful life
Wearout.

The discussion of the three life periods contained in the section on electronic reliability applies to device reliability as well.

1.8 Optimizing Device Reliability

Reliability optimization involves consideration of each of the life cycle periods. Major factors that influence and degrade a system's operational reliability must be addressed during design in order to control and maximize system reliability. Early failures may be eliminated by a systematic process of controlled screening and burn-in of components, assemblies and the device. Stress-related failures are minimized by providing adequate design margins for each component and the device as a whole. Wearout failures may be eliminated by conducting timely preventive maintenance on the device, with appropriate replacement of affected components.

1.9 Reliability's Effect on Medical Devices

Subjecting a medical device to a reliability program provides a structured approach to the product development process. It provides techniques that both improve the quality of the device over a period of time and reduce development and redevelopment time and cost. It yields statistical data that quantifies the success, or lack of success, of the development process and predicts future performance. It also assures that regulatory requirements are satisfied and gives confidence that regulatory inspections will produce no major discrepancies.

The use of the various reliability techniques results in decreased warranty costs and the resultant increase in customer acceptance. This enhances customer perception of the manufacturer and leads to a resultant increase in market share. Reliability techniques also reduce the risk of liability by assuring safety has been the primary concern during the design and development process. By reducing up-front costs, limiting liability risks and increasing future profits, implementation of a well-defined reliability assurance program is the basis of the success of any company.

1.10 Summary

Reliability is an important topic in the medical device field. Reliability concerns itself not only with the specified operation of a device, but also the safety of that device. Reliability affects the system specification, design, tolerances, safety margins, component choice, operation, maintenance and spare parts inventory. Reliability has many benefits, including decreased warranty costs, increased customer acceptance, enhanced customer image and thus a more profitable bottom line. It also helps in diminishing the risk of liability.

Before we discuss the basics of a reliability program, we need to understand the concept of failure and how this concept is an integral part of reliability.

1.11 References

1. Dhillon, B. S., *Reliability Engineering in Systems Design and Operation*. New York: Van Nostrand Reinhold Company, 1983.

2. Goldberg, M. F. and J. Vaccaro, editors. *Physics of Failure in Electronics*. Spartan Books, Inc., 1963.

3. Kececioglu, D., "Lecture Notes of AME-518 - Reliability Testing." University of Arizona, 1984.

4. Langer, E. and J. Meltroft, editors. *Reliability in Electrical and Electronic Components and Systems.* North Holland Publishing Company, 1982.

5. Lloyd, D. K. and M. Lipow, *Reliability Management, Methods and Mathematics.* 2nd Edition, Milwaukee, Wisconsin: The American Society for Quality Control, 1984.

6. MIL-STD-721C, *Definition of Terms for Reliability and Maintainability.* Washington, DC: Department of Defense, 1981.

7. O'Connor, P. D. T. *Practical Reliability Engineering.* New York: John Wiley and Sons, 1984.

8. Reliability Analysis Center. *Reliability Design Handbook.* Chicago: ITT Research Institute, 1975.

9. Sandberg, J. B. "Reliability For Profit . . . Not Just Regulation," *Quality Progress.* August, 1987.

2

Reliability and the Concept of Failure

Reliability is concerned with failures and their elimination. To understand what a failure is, we must first understand what an accepted operation is and what the accepted limits of that acceptance are. For example, if a medical device is subjected to a burst of electromagnetic interference and the software momentarily stops working, is that a failure? It depends on the application of the device and how it has been specified. If the software has been specified to detect the interference and gracefully shut the system down, notifying the user what is happening, the halt in operation is not a failure. If the software has been specified to continue working through a burst of interference, then the halt in operation is a failure.

The two examples show the difference in the breadth of acceptable operation. In the first case, the area of acceptable operation is wide, including a graceful shutdown of the system. In the second case, the area of acceptable operation is narrow. For any medical device, the area of acceptable operation must be clearly defined, based upon the intended application, the environment in which it is to be used and the product specification. Only after this area of acceptable operation is defined can the area of failure be established. This may be visualized as the graph in Figure 2.1.

The graph show a middle area denoted as "acceptable". Operation within this area is accepted as meeting the specification limits. Operation that falls outside these limits is classified as a failure.

2.1 Closely Related Terms

The term failure is closely related to other terms with which it is sometimes confused. These include:

Defect
Deficiency
Fault
Malfunction.

"Defect" indicates any imperfection, flaw, lack of completeness or other conditions at variance with technical requirements. It denotes such things as the unsatisfactory packaging of hardware, as well as part and equipment discrepancies, which may be responsible for failure.

"Deficiency" is a general term covering any defect, discrepancy or lack of conformance to specifications.

"Fault" is the immediate cause of a failure, such as maladjustment or misalignment.

"Malfunction" refers to any occurrence of unsatisfactory performance. It need not constitute a failure if readjustment of operator controls can restore an acceptable operating condition.

Figure 2.1 Graph of Acceptance Limits

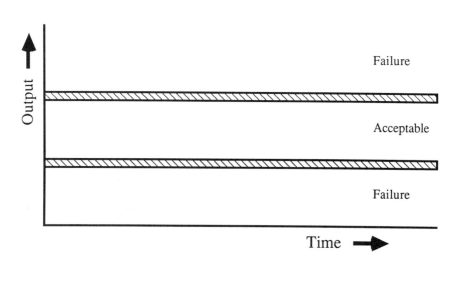

2.2 Failure

The term "failure" refers to the degradation of the performance of a device outside a specified value. It may be defined as:

The inability of a component or device to continue to perform its intended function.

This definition assumes the intended function of the component or device has been defined, so that deviation from the intended function may be established as a failure. The definition also assumes there must be a cause of the inability to perform the intended function. This cause must be the focal point for any type of failure analysis activity. Too often, "band-aids" are applied to device failures in an effort to get a quick fix. These may cause a temporary return to intended function, but eventually will fail because the real cause of the failure was not analyzed and corrected.

Failure must be precisely defined in practice. Care must be taken to assure that the failure criteria are not ambiguous. A failure must always be related to a measurable parameter or a clear indication. Defects, e.g., changes in appearance or minor degradation, which do not affect function, are not relevant to reliability.

2.3 Time Related Failures

There are three types of time related failures:

Early failures
Chance or random failures
Wearout failures.

2.3.1 Early Failures

Early failures occur usually within the first 1000 hours of operation. That is why integrated circuits, for example, are subjected to an accelerated burn-in at high temperature, equivalent to 1000 hours of operation. This is considered the industry standard for eliminating early failures. There are several causes for early failures:

Insufficient design debugging
Substandard components
Poor quality control
Poor manufacturing techniques
Poor workmanship
Insufficient burn-in
Improper installation
Replacing field components with non-screened ones.

2.3.2 Chance Failures

Chance or random failures occur during the useful life of the device. They are usually the hardest failures to duplicate and analyze. Causes of such failures include:

> Interference or overlap of designed-in strength
> Insufficient safety factors
> Occurrence of higher than expected random loads
> Occurrence of lower than expected random strengths
> Component defects
> Errors in usage
> Abuse.

2.3.3 Wearout Failures

Wearout failures occur at the end of the life cycle of a device or electronic component, or continuously throughout the life of a mechanical component. Causes of wearout failures include:

> Aging
> Wear
> Degradation in strength
> Creep
> Fatigue
> Corrosion
> Poor service or maintenance.

2.4 Operational Failures

Operational failures are described by the suddeness of the failure and whether the component or the device is able to return to its specified operation. For many products, failure is catastrophic. For others, performance degrades slowly and there is no clear end of life. Operational failures are classifed as:

> Catastrophic
> Drift
> Degradation
> Intermittent.

2.4.1 Catastrophic Failure

A catastrophic failure (Figure 2.2) occurs when a component or device suddenly fails and its output either goes to zero or occassionally to a very high level outside of the desirable performance limits.

Figure 2.2 Catastrophic Failure

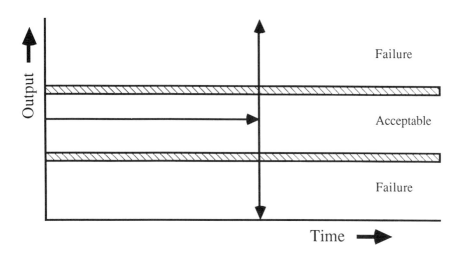

2.4.2 Drift Failure

A drift failure (Figure 2.3) occurs when the output steadily decreases or increases and eventually goes below the lower specification limit or above the upper specification limit. If the power is turned off and then back on again, the output comes back to within the successful performance limits and continues to operate within these limits.

2.4.3 Degradation Failure

A degradation failure (Figure 2.4) occurs when the output goes below the specified performance limit. If the power is turned off and after a rest period it is turned on, the output level will come back to the level it was prior to the power being turned off and then continues to degrade.

2.4.4 Intermittent Failure

An intermittent failure (Figure 2.5) occurs when, at an unknown time and for an unknown reason, the output goes to zero and then suddenly comes back on again to specified performance limits. This type of failure is difficult to correct.

Figure 2.3 Drift Failure

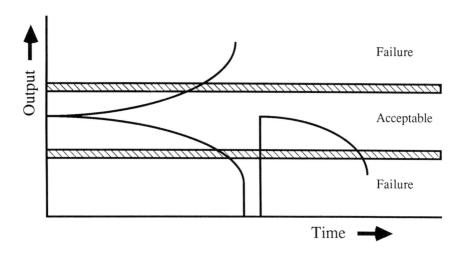

Figure 2.4 Degradation Failure

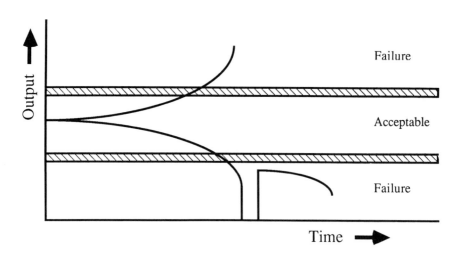

Figure 2.5 Intermittent Failure

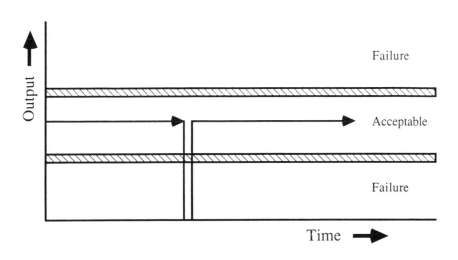

2.5 Reliability Parameters

Failures are related to various reliability parameters including:

Failure rate
Mean Time Between Failure (MTBF)
Reliability.

2.5.1 Failure Rate

The failure rate of a component or device is the probability of failure per unit of time for the items still functioning. The best estimate of the failure rate is given by the equation:

$$\lambda = r/t$$

where λ is the failure rate
r is the number of failures
t is the accumulated operating time
of the item

Failure rate is normally expressed in failures per million hours. Documents, such as MIL-HDBK-217, list all component failure rates with this notation. Such documents, in listing failure rates make the assumption that the component is in its useful life period (constant failure rate, exponential distribution). For a component in its useful life period, the failure rate is the reciprocal of the Mean Time Between Failure (MTBF).

2.5.2 Mean Time Between Failure

The Mean Time Between Failure (MTBF) is defined as the mean value of the length of time between consecutive failures, computed as the ratio of the cumulative observed time to the number of failures under stated conditions. MTBF is the parameter primarily used for comparison of devices, the one with the greater MTBF being more reliable.

Practically, MTBF is the time in the life of the device or component when 63% of the devices currently in operation will have failed once. Once again, the assumption is made that the device is in its useful life period. There are several ways to calculate this parameter, depending on the way the data is obtained. These are discussed in detail in the chapter on data analysis.

2.5.3 Reliability

Reliability was defined earlier as the probability that a device will perform a required function, under specified conditions, for a specified period of time, at a desired confidence level. Practically, reliability is the percentage of devices currently in operation that will not fail during a specified mission time. As an example, a company may decide that, in order for a medical monitor to be a successful product, it must have a reliability of .995 for an operating time of three years. This means that after three years of operation, 99.5% of the units will have experienced no failures.

A similar example can be given from the aerospace industry. A rocket carrying a space shuttle into orbit would only have to operate for a period of five minutes or less to accomplish its purpose. Because of the lives of the astronauts on board the shuttle, the safety of launch observers and the cost of the shuttle and rocket, it must operate without failure every time it is fired. Therefore a reliability of 0.99999999999 for a period of five minutes operation is not an unreasonable reliability specification for the rocket. Calculation of the reliability parameter is discussed in detail in the chapter on data analysis.

2.6 Failure Correction

The term "repair" refers to all actions performed as a result of failure to restore the device to a specified condition. Repair relies on a meaningful failure analysis procedure to identify the *cause* of the failure and establish a resolution for it. Repair may include any or all of the following activities:

Localization
Isolation
Disassembly
Interchange
Reassembly
Alignment
Checkout
Calibration.

This subject is discussed further in the chapter on field operation.

2.7 Summary

The primary element of reliability is failure. Failures are unique to each individual medical device, based upon complexity, intended application and the environment in which it is used. The occurrence of failures allow the calculation of various reliability parameters, which indicate how good the device is and how it compares to similar devices, both its predecessors and its competitors. The philosophy of reliability is to design out failures and take steps to prevent their occurrence. This philosophy is promoted in the many domestic and international device standards currently in effect.

2.8 References

1. Dhillon, B. S., *Reliability Engineering in System Design and Operation*. New York: Van Nostrand Reinhold Company, 1983.

2. Goldberg, M. F. and J. Vaccaro, editors. *Physics of Failure in Electronics*. Spartan Books, Inc., 1963.

3. Kececioglu, D., "Lecture Notes of AME-518 - Reliability Testing." University of Arizona, 1984.

4. Lloyd, D. K. and M. Lipow, *Reliability Management, Methods and Mathematics*. 2nd Edition. Milwaukee, Wisconsin: The American Society for Quality Control, 1984.

5. MIL-HDBK-217, *Reliability Prediction of Electronic Equipment.* Washington, DC: Department of Defense, 1986.

6. MIL-STD-721C, *Definition of Terms for Reliability and Maintainability.* Washington, DC: Department of Defense, 1981.

3

Reliability, Standards and Regulations

Medical devices are subject to evolving demands throughout the world. Competition demands the product comply with the ever changing requirements of increasingly sophisticated markets and rapid technological developments. An integral part of the design process is conformance to the product disciplines, which make up the world of standards·and regulations. An added concern is liability. The cost of product related injuries, as reflected in court judgements and insurance premiums, has climbed dramatically in recent years, making product safety and reliability the cornerstones of medical device design.

Any electromechanical device is subject to standards and regulations to assure safe and reliable operation. The purpose of a standard or regulation is to provide manufacturers and users with a method of assuring a product is safe for the patient, safe for the user and performs according to its stated specifications. The standards address such issues as electrical safety, leakage current, safety testing, performance standards and manufacturing requirements. The additional regulations govern sale and distribution of a device in a country. Figure 3.1 is a summary of applicable medical device standards in the United States and in other countries.

In most countries, the applicable product safety standards and regulations must be complied with before the device can be marketed. In the United States, the Food and Drug Administration is charged with assuring that medical devices are safe, effective and reliable for their intended use.

3.1 Food and Drug Administration (FDA)

In 1906, the FDA enacted its first regulations addressing public health. While these regulations did not address medical devices per se, they did establish a foundation for future regulations. It was not until 1938, with

Figure 3.1 Selected Standards Organizations

UNITED STATES	REST OF WORLD
American National Standards Institute	Association Francaise de Normalisation Tour Europe
American Society for Testing Materials	British Standards Institute
Association for Advancement of Medical Instrumentation	Canadian Standards Institute
City of Chicago	Department of Health and Social Services
City of Los Angeles	Deutsches Institut fur Normung
Food and Drug Administration	European Committee for Electrotechnical Standardization
Institute of Electrical and Electronic Engineers	International Electrotechnical Commission
Instrument Society of America	International Organization for Standardization
Joint Commission on Accreditation of Healthcare Organizations	Japanese Standards Association
National Fire Protection Association	Technischer Überwachungs-Verein
Underwriters Laboratory	Verband Deutscher Elektrotechniker

the passage of the Federal Food, Drug and Cosmetic Act (FFD&C), that the FDA was authorized, for the first time, to regulate medical devices. This act provided for regulation of adulterated or misbranded drugs, cosmetics and devices that were entered into interstate commerce. The act required only premarket approval for drugs and cosmetics. A medical device could be marketed without being federally reviewed and approved.

In the years following World War II, the FDA focused much of its attention on drugs and cosmetics. Over-the-counter drugs became regulated in 1951. In 1962, the FDA began requesting safety and efficacy data on new drugs and cosmetics.

By the mid-1960s, it became clear that the provisions of the FFD&C Act were not adequate to regulate the complex medical devices of the times to assure both patient and user safety. Thus, a study group, the Cooper Committee, was formed in 1969 to examine the problems associated with medical devices and to develop concepts for new regulations. This group recommended that future device regulation follow a three-tiered system:

> One class for devices that would essentially be exempt from premarket approval and performance standards
>
> A second class for devices that would require premarket approval and compliance with quality assurance and performance standards
>
> A third class, intended particularly for life-support devices, that would require premarket approval, compliance with quality assurance and performance standards, as well as providing safety and efficacy information.

In devising this system, the committee aimed to balance public safety concerns with industry fears about the burdens of regulation.

In 1976, with input from the Cooper Committee, the FDA created the Medical Device Amendments to the FFD&C Act, which were subsequently signed into law. The purpose of the amendments was to assure that medical devices were safe, effective and properly labeled for their intended use. To accomplish this mandate, the amendments provided the FDA with the authority to regulate devices during most phases of their development, testing, production, distribution and use. This marked the first time the FDA clearly distinguished between devices and drugs.

A medical device was defined as:

> Any instrument, apparatus or other similar or related article, including component, part or accessory, which is intended for use in the diagnosis of disease or other conditions, or in the cure, mitigation, treatment or prevention of disease, in man or other animals.

Regulatory requirements were derived from this 1976 law. Medical devices are divided into three classes with regulatory requirements based on the individual classes.

> Class I is defined as the class of devices that are subject to the general controls of the Federal Food, Drug and Cosmetic Act including premarket notification, registration and list-

ing, prohibitions against adulteration and misbranding and rules for good manufacturing practices.

Class II is defined as the class of devices that are or eventually will be subject to the requirements of a performance standard in addition to the requirements of Class I.

Class III is defined as the class of devices for which premarket approval is or will be required. Devices in this class are generally life-sustaining or life-supporting devices.

In 1978, with the authority granted the FDA by the amendments, the Good Manufacturing Practices (GMP) were promulgated. The GMP represents a quality assurance program intended to control the manufacturing, packaging, storage, distribution and installation of medical devices. This regulation was intended to allow only safe and effective devices to reach the market place. It is this regulation that has the greatest effect on the medical device industry. It allows the FDA to inspect a company's operations and take action on any noted deficiencies, including prohibition of device shipment. The GMP is examined in more detail in the chapter on reliability in manufacturing.

Recent regulations specific to medical devices are the Medical Device Reporting (MDR) regulation of 1984 and the Device Reconditioner/Rebuilder (DRR) regulation of 1988. The FDA used the authority granted by the complaint handling portion of the GMP to enact the MDR regulation. This regulation mandated that a device manufacturer or distributor notify the FDA of any complaint involving a patient injury or death. The DRR requires that a firm that acquires ownership of used devices, refurbishes them and then commercially distributes them is subject to many of the provisions of the regulations that affect the original device manufacturers, such as the MDA, GMP and MDR.

Recently, the FDA has concentrated much of its attention on the regulation of medical device software. A draft policy was published for comment in September, 1987. To date, a final policy has not been published. While there is currently no regulation addressing this area, the FDA is conducting portions of its inspections of devices and firms as if this proposed regulation was in effect. They have held training courses for their inspectors on computers and software and have published inspection guidelines on the subject. We will discuss the FDA and software in more detail in the chapter on reliable software design.

The FDA is currently looking at possible regulations that would require hospitals, nursing homes and ambulatory surgical facilities to notify the FDA of any patient injuries and deaths resulting from the use of medical devices.

3.2 Basic Standards Organizations

There are four basic standards for medical devices upon which all others are based. They are general electrical safety standards for medical devices and include:

Standard	Year of Implementation
UL 544	1972
IEC 601	1979
NFPA 99 (formerly 76B)	1982
CSA C22.2	1984

Of the four standards, there are no major differences between UL, CSA and NFPA. IEC is less stringent for leakage current, but more stringent on design processes. An important observation is that the UL 544 standard was implemented prior to the Medical Device Amendments. It is also important to note that while the UL standard is voluntary, the CSA and IEC standards are mandatory.

There are many standards and standards testing facilities similar to UL. These include:

Canadian Standards Association (CSA)
National Fire Protection Association (NFPA)
City of Los Angeles
City of Chicago
City of Detroit
Illinois Institute of Technology Research Institute (IITRI)
Electronic Testing Laboratories (ETL).

There are many standards and testing facilities similar to IEC. These include:

Deutsches Institut fur Normung (Germany)
Verband Deutscher Elektrotechniker (Germany)
British Standards Institute (United Kingdom)
Technischer Überwachungs-Verein (Germany)
Japanese Industrial Standards (Japan).

There are also may countries which have their own individual interpretations of the IEC standard. These include:

Finland (Suomen Standardisoimisliitto)
France (Association Francaise de Normalisation)
Sweden (Swedish Planning and Rationalization Institute for the Health and Social Services)
Spain (Instituto Espanol de Normalization)
Most other members of the European Economic Community.

It would take a book in itself to cover all the various standards applicable to medical devices. For our purposes we will review only the major ones.

3.2.1 Underwriters Laboratory (UL)

Underwriters Laboratory is an independent, not for profit testing laboratory organized for the purpose of investigating materials, devices, products, equipment construction, methods and systems with respect to hazards affecting life and property. It tests devices in six different areas:

Burglary Protection and Signaling
Casualty and Chemical Hazards
Electrical
Fire Protection
Heating, Air Conditioning and Refrigeration
Marine.

UL inspection services personnel visit companies unannounced to verify that products that bear the UL mark comply with applicable UL safety requirements. The registered UL mark on a device is a means by which a manufacturer, distributor or importer can show that samples of the product have been verified for compliance with safety standards.

Many hospitals require that the medical devices they purchase comply with applicable UL standards. If the devices do not comply, they are not purchased.

3.2.2 International Electrotechnical Commission (IEC)

The International Electrotechnical Commission, based in Geneva, Switzerland, was founded in 1906. It is the authority for world standards for electrical and electronic engineering. The council of the IEC is the governing body that consists of presidents of the national committees for 42 countries.

The objective of IEC is to promote international cooperation on all questions of standardizations in the fields of electrical and electronic engineering. It issues publications, including recommendations for international standards, which the national committees are expected to use in international standards. The IEC standards are the basis for national standards in over 100 countries.

IEC also promotes safety, compatibility, interchangeability and acceptability. It helps manufacturers, distributors and users of electrical and electronic goods and services at all levels, worldwide.

3.2.3 Canadian Standards Association (CSA)

The Canadian Standards Association is a membership association that brings people and ideas together to develop services that meet the needs of businesses, industry, governments and consumers. Among the many services available are standards development, testing and application of the CSA mark to certified products, testing to international standards, worldwide inspection and related services.

CSA develops concensus standards in eight major program fields:

> Lifestyles and the Environment
> Electrical/Electronic
> Communications/Information
> Construction
> Energy
> Transportation/Distribution
> Materials Technology
> Production Management Systems.

CSA has four main operating divisions and two staff divisions. It has several types of certification including model, line, combined engineering and category. It also has facilities for testing to such international standards as:

> International Electrochemical Commission (IEC)
> British Standards Institute (BSI)
> Standards Association of Australia (SAA)
> Verband Deutscher Elektrotechniker (VDE).

3.2.4 National Fire Protection Association (NFPA)

The National Fire Protection Association is organized to assure the appointment of technically competent committees, with balanced representation, to establish criteria to minimize the hazards of fire, explosion and electricity in health care facilities. These criteria include:

Performance
Maintenance
Testing
Safe practices
Material
Equipment
Appliances.

The NFPA does not approve, inspect or certify any installation, procedure, equipment or material. NFPA has no authority to police or en-
force compliance to their standards. However, installations may base acceptance of a device on compliance with their standards.

3.3 Other Standards Organizations

3.3.1 Association for the Advancement of Medical Instrumentation (AAMI)

The Association for the Advancement of Medical Instrumentation is an
alliance of health care professional, united by the common goal of increasing the understanding and beneficial use of medical devices and
instrumentation. In meeting this goal, AAMI distributes information
in the form of various publications, including voluntary standards.

AAMI is a highly respected and widely recognized national and international consensus standards organization. AAMI is accredited by
the American National Standards Institute (ANSI) and is one of the prin-
cipal voluntary standards organizations in the world.

3.3.2 British Standards Institute (BSI)

The British Standards Institute is the United Kingdom's main national
standards organization. BSI has developed a Registered Firm System
that rates a company's ability to provide high-quality products and services. This is based on British Standard 5750 - Quality Systems. This
standard defines how a total quality system can be implemented to assure that all performance requirements of the customer are fully met.
Registered firms must have a documented quality system that complies
with the appropriate part of BS5750 and the relevant technical sched-
ule. The companies are inspected to verify compliance.

The principles included in preparing British standards are:

They must satisfy a generally recognized demand
They must meet the needs of the economy
They must consider the interests of producers and users.

BSI has established an international reputation, with many of its standards having been adopted by other countries. It also represents the United Kingdom in the International Organization for Standardization (ISO) and the IEC.

3.3.3 International Special Committee on Radio Interference (CISPR)

The International Special Committe on Radio Interference is a committee under the auspices of the IEC and run through a Plenary Assembly consisting of delegates from all the member bodies, including the United States. The committee is headquartered in Geneva, Switzerland and is composed of seven subcommittees, including:

> Radio Interference Measurement and Statistical Methods
> Interference from Industrial, Scientific and Medical Radio Frequency Apparatus
> Interference from Overhead Power Lines, High Voltage Equipment and Electric Traction Systems
> Interference Related to Motor Vehicles and Internal Combustion Engines
> Interference Characteristics of Radio Receivers
> Interference from Motor, Household Appliances, Lighting Apparatus and the like
> Interference from Information Technology Equipment.

3.3.4 Department of Health (DOH)

The Department of Health has the same responsibility in the United Kingdom that the FDA has in the United States. DOH sets forth standards for medical devices and has established a Good Manufacturing Practice for Medical Equipment, similar to that of the FDA. DOH is headquartered in London and currently has reciprocity with the FDA of GMP inspections for non-sterile medical devices. FDA will accept DOH inspection data as their own and DOH will accept FDA inspection data.

3.3.5 European Committee for Standardization (CEN)

The European Committee for Standardization is the regional body active in areas other than the electronic interests of CENELAC. CEN is headquartered in Brussels, Belgium and is composed of sixteen members, twelve of whom come from the European Economic Community.

CEN performs an important role in the harmonization of non-electrical standards in Europe.

3.3.6 European Committee for Electrotechnical Standardization (CENELAC)

The European Committee for Electrotechnical Standardization is a private organization serving a regional, rather than a national standardization function. Headquartered in Brussels, Belgium it is composed of seventeen members, twelve of whom are from the European Economic Community. CENELAC's aims are to remove technical barriers to trade, which result from conflicting requirements of the technical content of the national electrotechnical standards of its members. It bases most of its standards on those of IEC. A separate Mark Committee within CENELAC deals with the problem of recognition of national marks of conformity in separate countries.

3.3.7 Institute of Electrical and Electronic Engineers (IEEE)

The Institute of Electrical and Electronic Engineers was founded in 1884 and is one of the oldest societies in the U.S. It is an organization that develops standards on a variety of topics relating to electrical and electronic equipment. In recent years, a primary focus for the standards organization has been the areas of software development and software quality assurance. Some of their software standards have been accredited by the American National Standards Institute and have been used primarily for the development and validation of military software. Recently, these standards have been referenced by the FDA in the development of guidelines on medical software.

3.3.8 International Organization for Standardization (ISO)

The International Organization for Standardization is the specialized international agency for standardization. Its members are the national standards organizations of 89 countries.

The scope of ISO technical work extends to all fields of standardization, with the exception of electrical and electronic engineering which, by agreement, are the responsibility of IEC. The ISO publishes international standards.

The ISO consists of 162 technical committees and some 600 subcommittees that are organized and supported by technical secretariats in 32 countries. The Central Secretariat in Geneva, Switzerland, helps coordinate ISO operations, administers voting and approval procedures and publishes the international standards.

ISO coordinates the exchange of information on international and national standards, technical regulations and other standards-type documents through an information network, called ISONET, which links the ISO Information Center in Geneva with similar national centers in over 50 countries.

3.3.9 Japanese Standards Association (JSA)

The unified national system of industrial standardization began to function by the setup of the Japanese Engineering Standards Committee (JESC) in 1921. This group undertook the establishment of national standards. In 1949, the Industrial Standardization Law was promulgated and the Japanese Industrial Standards Committee (JISC) was established under the law as an advisory organization of competent ministers in charge of the elaboration of Japanese Industrial Standards (JIS) and the designation of the JIS mark to products.

The Japanese Standards Association was established as a public institution for the promotion of industrial standardization on December 6, 1945, under government authorization. JSA has no true performance standards, but tends to follow IEC 601-1. JSA does have a complicated approval process that can be very lengthy (up to 9 months). This process can delay distribution of products in Japan. JSA activities include:

> Standards and document publishing
> Seminars and consulting services
> Research on standardization
> National sales agent for foreign national standard bodies.

3.4 Contacting the Organizations

Addresses and telephone numbers of major standards and regulatory organizations are listed in Appendix 3.

3.5 European Harmonization

The European Community (EC) is a grouping of twelve Western European countries established in 1957. The community is made up of the following member states:

> Belgium
> Denmark
> France
> Greece

Ireland
Italy
Luxembourg
Netherlands
Portugal
Spain
United Kingdom
West Germany

Most European member countries have their own standards and laws reflecting quality and safety practices in their national home markets. These are drawn up by national standard bodies such as the British Standards Institute (United Kingdom), Association Francaise de Normalisation (France), Technischer Uberwachungs-Verein (Germany) and Swedish Planning and Rationalization Institute for the Health and Social Services (Sweden). National standards are a serious barrier to trade when different standards apply in each country and when members do not recognize other arrangements for testing and certifying products to assure they satisfy national or European standards.

The purpose of the European Community was to create a common market free of internal barriers to trade. After 32 years of effort, however, the market is still segmented. The goal of the 1992 program is to establish a single market within the European community by removing barriers to trade. The market would consist of a total population of 323 million people, approximately 100 million more than the United States and 200 million more than Japan. Despite the larger population, the EC would trail the United States in gross national product.

In order to achieve this goal, representatives of each country have been developing a directive to guide the development of this market. The directive includes the following objectives:

> Member states shall take all necessary steps to ensure that devices are placed on the market only if their design and manufacture are such that they will not impair patient and operator safety when properly used and maintained according to the purposes intended.

> Devices shall satisfy the essential safety requirements including protection against electrical, mechanical, thermal, radiation and energy-related hazards.

> Member states shall not on their territory impede the placing on the market and the circulation and use of devices bearing the mark of approval (CE).

The creation of a single market involves harmonization in two areas: the general business environment (taxation, business law, transfer of capital, etc.) and elimination of technical barriers to trade related to the safety of products. The latter will effect the medical device industry and its impact will be significant. 1992 should be seen as a specific milestone in a larger process of remodeling the business environment of Europe.

3.5.1 Regulatory Institutions

The EC has established institutions that mimic the normal western governmental system of executive, legislative and judicial functions. These institutions include:

> the Commission
> the Council
> the European Parliament
> the European Court of Justice
> the European Standards Organizations.

3.5.1.1 The Commission

The Commission is the executive arm of the European Community. It is responsible for initiating Community policies, drafting legislation and assuring the proper application and enforcement of Community legislation.

The Commission is composed of 17 members, 2 from each of the 5 largest member countries and 1 each from the other seven. Members are appointed for renewable 4-year terms by common agreement of the member governments.

3.5.1.2 The Council

The Council is the decision-making body of the European Community. It is reponsible for adopting or rejecting legislative proposals submitted by the Commission. It is also responsible for taking broad policy decisions which may then be transformed into specific legislative proposals by the Commission.

The Council is composed of ministers or government level representatives of the 12 member countries. The membership varies with the subjects to be discussed at individual Council meetings.

3.5.1.3 The European Parliament

The European Parliament is composed of 518 members directly elected by citizens of the European Community member countries. The Parliament meets in plenary session once each month.

The Parliament is responsible to supervise the activities of the Commission and the Council and to render its opinion on all proposals for European Community legislation. The Parliament is also responsible for adopting the European Community annual budget.

3.5.1.4 The European Court of Justice

The European Court of Justice has the responsibility to interpret and apply European Community law. The decisions of the Court may not be appealed.

The Court is composed of 13 judges appointed for 6-year renewable terms by agreement among member countries.

3.5.2 Regulatory Schemes

The objectives of the regulations are twofold:

> Provide a harmonized regulatory procedure to replace individual national systems

> Provide a mark of approval (CE) so that the CE mark gained in one country will guarantee free distribution throughout all member countries.

The regulatory schemes for medical devices will consists of:

> Directives which specify the legal requirements for medical devices

> Harmonized technical standards which specify what the requirements mean in practice

> Conformity assessment modules which indicate how regulatory compliance will be controlled.

Good Manufacturing Practices regulations are based on ISO 9000 and the four medical device classifications:

Classification	GMP Regulation
Active implantables	ISO 9000-1
Active medical devices	ISO 9000-1
Non-active medical devices	ISO 9000-2
In vitro diagnostics	ISO 9000-3

Figure 3.2 Proposed product approval process

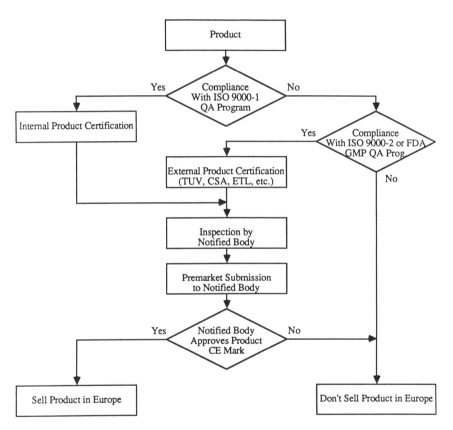

Certification will include design, manufacture and testing to
comply with standards addressing the following areas.

Good Manufacturing Practices (ISO 9000)
Product Effectiveness
Electrical Safety (IEC 601-1)
Electromagnetic Compatibility
Clinical Research
Biocompatibility
Radiation Safety
Labelling
Components
Software

The proposed product approval process (Figure 3.2) uses either internal or external product certification based on compliance with either ISO 9000-1 or 9000-2.

3.5.3 Medical Device Classification

Four working groups have been establishged to draft medical device directives. The working groups correspond to the four divisions of medical products:

> Active implantable electromedical devices, consisting of permanently implanted electromedical devices which use electricity from an implanted battery or an external power source. Examples include pacemakers and neural stimulators.

> Active medical devices, consisting of external electromedical equipment. Examples include monitoring and imaging devices.

> Non-active medical devices consisting of sterile hospital products and other medical devices not covered by the other groups. An example of a device from this group would be electrodes.

> *In vitro* diagnostic products.

3.5.4 European Free Trade Area

Another group of countries, the European Free Trade Area (EFTA) is currently reviewing options for integration with the European Community. Some members may eventually join the EC. EFTA member states are:

> Austria
> Finland
> Iceland
> Norway
> Sweden
> Switzerland

3.6 Summary

Medical standards exist to help assure medical devices are safe and effective for their intended use. Some are voluntary, others are mandatory. Some customers require compliance with certain standards prior to purchasing medical equipment. Country standards also exist as requirements to be satisfied before selling and distributing devices in that country. The development of the European Community will strive to provide uniform standards and regulations for European distribution.

Standards require additional effort in the design and development process in order to satisfy their requirements. It is more cost effective to be aware of the requirements prior to beginning the design so the requirements may be incorporated early in the design, rather than as an afterthought.

3.7 References

1. Booz-Allen and Hamilton, *1992 Harmonization: A Survey of European Chief Executives*. London: Pauline-George Processing, 1988.

2. Bureau of Medical Devices, Office of Small Manufacturers Assistance, *Regulatory Requirements for Marketing a Device*. U.S. Department of Health and Human Services, 1982.

3. Canadian Standards Association, *One Step Guide—Your Roadmap for Getting Help When You Need It*. Canadian Standards Association, 1985.

4. Center for Devices and Radiological Health, *Device Good Manufacturing Practices Manual*. Washington DC: U.S. Department of Health and Human Services, 1987.

5. Commission of the European Communities, *Draft Proposal for a Council Directive Relating to Active Medical Devices*. Brussels, Belgium, 12 May, 1989.

6. Dash, G. and I. Straus, "The ABC's of Regulations and Standards," *Compliance Engineering*. 1989 Reference Guide.

7. Food and Drug Administration, *Federal Food, Drug, and Cosmetic Act, As Amended, January 1979*. Washington DC: U.S. Government Printing Office, 1979.

8. Kyper, C. H., "The 510(k) Route to the Marketplace," *Medical Device and Diagnostic Industry*. January, 1982.

9. McBride, S. et al, *The Guide to Biomedical Standards*. Brea, California: Quest Publishing Company, 1989.

10. Medical Technology Consultants Europe Ltd., *An Introduction to the European Community and the 1992 Single Market.* Medical Technology Consultants Europe Ltd., 1989.

11. Mori, G., "The Japanese Standards Association (JSA)—Its Role in the Standardization Activity in Japan," *ASTM Standardization News.* October, 1987.

12. NFPA, *NFPA 99 Health Care Facilities 1987 Edition.* National Fire Protection Agency, 1987.

13. Office of Standards and Regulations, *Medical Devices Standards Activities Report.* Washington, DC: U.S. Department of Health and Human Services, 1987.

14. Oppenheimer, Wolff and Donnelly, *An Overview of the European Community's 1992 Program.* Washington, DC, 1988.

15. Underwriters Laboratory, *Submitting Products to Underwriters Laboratories Incorporated.* 1985.

16. Unknown, "International Standards—It's a Small World After All," *Quality,* August, 1986.

17. 21 CFR 7

18. 21 CFR 803

19. 21 CFR 820

4

Overview of the Product Development Process

New products create profit and growth if they are successful; disaster if they are not. To be successful, a project development process must meet certain corporate objectives, namely customer satisfaction and financial return.

The primary objective of a product development process is the selection, development and introduction, at the lowest possible cost, of a safe, effective and reliable device that:

Will make a contribution to the market
Can be efficiently manufactured
Can be successfully sold and supported.

The product development process consists of various phases necessary to assure the product that is developed is safe, effective and reliable. In every case, the process requires the cooperation of: Design Engineering, Marketing, Manufacturing, Reliability Assurance, Regulatory Affairs, Quality Assurance and Customer Service. Although all groups may not be active at any particular time, each will be involved throughout the process. Some companies have formed a project development team, with the Marketing representative as the Product Manager and the leading Design Engineer as the Product Development Manager. The project team meets at regular intervals, determined by the current activity. Minutes of team meetings are documented and become part of the product file.

The advantage of the project team approach is that each member has input into the development of the product. For example, the Manufacturing representative can assure the design is manufacturable and the Service representative that the design is serviceable early in the development process. This prevents project delays later to correct problems.

The typical product development cycle (Figure 4.1) consists of six stages necessary for a reliable device:

>Feasibility
>Design
>Validation
>Manufacturing
>Field operation
>Feedback.

A general overview of each phase is included below and is discussed in detail in the following chapters.

Figure 4.1 Product Life Cycle

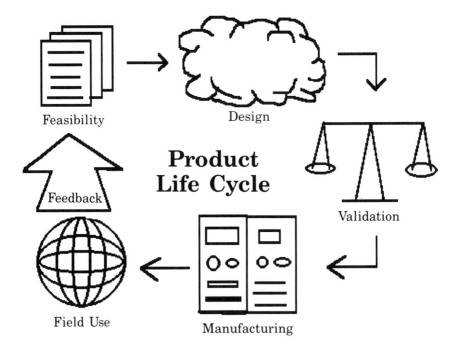

4.1 Feasibility

The first step in the development process is defining the new product. Preliminary information is gathered through marketing and customer surveys. Once the preliminary data is collected, a Product Specification is written, with the approval of the appropriate development team members. Some of the product parameters specified in the Product Specification are:

> Type of product
> The market it addresses
> Function of the unit
> Product parameters
> Accuracy requirements
> Required tolerances
> Anticipated enviroment
> Anticipated misuse
> Life of the product
> Reliability goal
> Applicable standards
> Human factors
> Safety issues.

This specification becomes a controlled document, so that future changes are controlled by a revision control process. This approach assures all members of the team are aware of the changes and lets them approve them.

4.2 Design

Once the Product Specification is written, the Design Engineering team develops the System Specification, which details the product design. The specification includes:

> Hardware block diagram
> Technology to be used
> Software block diagram
> Hardware/software compatibility plan
> Required tolerances
> Standards requirements.

With regard to hardware, the design phase includes anticipation of and designing around misuse of the device, establishment of a reliability test plan, use of reliable design principles and selection of reliable components. A parts analysis, using MIL-HDBK-217, can determine, by looking at the failure rate of each component, whether the device will meet its reliability goal.

With regard to software, the design phase includes the establishment of a software specification, design of the program structure, and a design review prior to beginning coding.

The regulatory application submitted to the FDA, 510(k) or pre-market approval, is usually submitted during this phase, as soon as an engineering prototype has been evaluated and proven to be safe. This submission allows sufficient time for clinical testing and for the FDA to ask its questions and approve the device for distribution prior to it being marketed.

The 510(k) product approval is required for most Class I and all Class II medical devices. It requires moderate safety, efficacy, reliability and standards compliance studies. The approval is based on the manufacturer proving substantial equivalency of the proposed device to other approved devices or technologies. The 510(k) review usually takes 90 days to complete. Questions or incomplete data may extend the time period to approval.

The pre-market approval (PMA) is required for all Class III medical devices. It requires extensive safety, efficacy and reliability studies. Approximately 10-20% of all devices are approved in this manner. The approval is similar to new drug studies and requires clinical data to prove the safety, efficacy and reliability of the device. The PMA usually takes several years to complete and receive FDA approval.

4.3 Validation

Validation is a critical phase in the development of a product because it indicates how much reliability exists in the design. Reliability cannot be tested into a unit. Testing only indicates the degree of its presence or absence.

Hardware validation includes various types of tests depending on the intended use of the device. Hardware validation includes:

> Vendor Evaluation
> Component Verification
> Failure Mode and Effect Analysis.

Software validation begins with verifying the individual modules, integrating the modules and then combining the hardware and the software. These tests may include 1) the use of an emulator for error introduction to the individual modules, 2) varying the input power to to simulate a brown out and determine its effect on the software and 3) simulating anticipated misuse, such as dropping input cycles, releasing a burst of Rf energy in the area of the device or inputting a response in a way the software does not expect.

Product validation is the final chance to detect and remove problems before placing the device in a customer's hands. Product validation varies, based on intended use, but typically includes:

Environmental testing
Hardware/software compatibility
Safety evaluation
Clinical testing
Shipping tests
Standards evaluation
Reliability demonstration.

The validation phase closes with a review meeting in which all previous activity is discussed. Following successful completion of the review and receipt of FDA approval for the device, it is released to Manufacturing. It is important to realize that no matter how reliable the design has proven to be, the device must be manufactured reliably or it will not be a success.

4.4 Manufacturing

Once the design is released, it is placed under revision level control. Various production tasks then begin:

Production components are ordered
Incoming inspection files are developed for each component
Rejection procedures are established
Manufacturing processes and test procedures are developed
Test fixtures and burn-in apparatus are built and verified
Files for the Device History Records are made.

It is important that standards for all processes, such as soldering, component insertion and electrostatic discharge protection, are in place and being followed by all Manufacturing personnel. It is also important that each individual is his/her own quality inspector doing the best possible job and indicating when the quality of assemblies received is below acceptable levels.

Procedures for handling and evaluating components and assemblies that do not satisfy specifications must be established. Failure analysis of these components or assemblies will yield the necessary information to assess the problem and develop a solution. Failure analysis is also required by the Good Manufacturing Practices (GMP) regulation. Graphing of this data to provide a trend or history of the component or assembly will also provide a tool to monitor the manufacturing process.

Statistical Process Control (SPC) techniques help the overall quality and reliability of the manufacturing process. Records should be kept on individual processes to determine where problem areas are and suggest methods for improvement. Statistics should be kept on components or assemblies pre- and post-burn-in. The failure rate at final test should be constantly evaluated to assure the process is working correctly.

4.5 Field Operation

The device has finally made it through the design and manufacturing stages and is ready to ship to the customer. It carries the company name and reputation and if all activity has gone well, the unit should work well in the field. Two activities are important when dealing with field units:

> Preventive maintenance
> Customer service.

If sufficient reliability activity has been completed, components or assemblies with a good chance of early failure should be identified and the time of failure approximated. If this is done, establish a preventive maintenance program that indicates the component or assembly to be changed and a time to change it, prior to that indicated in the reliability parameters. This keeps the device operational and the customer satisfied.

Since medical devices are designed and manufactured by human beings, it is inevitable that, sooner or later, the device may experience a failure. When this happens, resolve the problem. Do not just apply a "band-aid" to get the unit operational. Analyze the problem, find the cause of the problem and resolve it. This approach makes customers happier than having the service representative living in their area. Of utmost importance is the documentation of the problem. This data can be used to calculate warranty costs and to provide information to the engineers in the office.

4.6 Feedback

This phase is the one most often ignored. The design or manufacturing engineers cannot work to resolve a field problem unless they know there is a problem. In order to facilitate this feedback, field problem reports should be filed for each service call. This report should include the following detail:

> Name of the device
> Serial number
> Date of service activity
> Symptom
> Diagnosis
> List of parts replaced
> Service Representative identification
> Number of labor hours required.

This data can then be entered in a database, with the addition of the manufacturing date, time since manufacturing and time since last service. The database then provides the means for sorting the data by manufacturing date, failure code and/or time since manufacturing. This data could also be used to monitor the effectiveness of each Service Representative, to monitor the labor time required per failure code and to assess the complexity of the design. From this information, decisions can be made about future revisions or future model changes. When this happens, the cycle begins again.

4.7 Summary

The life cycle of a product is a series of sequential activities which, when properly completed, provides the basis for a safe, effective, reliable and commercially successful product. The needs and desires of the customer will have been documented, the device designed, validated and manufactured to meet those requirements and the device shipped to the customer to satisfy those requirements. Complemented with an effective service plan, including proper feedback to the appropriate personnel, the customer can feel secure in the knowledge the device can be used to accomplish its intended application.

4.8 References

1. Dhillon, B. S., *Reliability Engineering in Systems Design and Operation*. New York: Van Nostrand Reinhold Company, 1983.

2. Lloyd, D. K. and M. Lipow, *Reliability Management, Methods and Mathematics*. 2nd Edition Milwaukee, Wisconsin: The American Society for Quality Control, 1984.

3. MIL-HDBK-217, *Reliability Prediction of Electronic Equipment.* Washington, DC: Department of Defense, 1986.

4. MIL-STD-785B, *Reliability Program for Systems and Equipment Development and Production.* Washington, DC: Department of Defense, 1980.

5. O'Connor, P. D. T., *Practical Reliability Engineering.* New York: John Wiley and Sons, 1984.

6. Oppenheimer, C. P., "Reliable Designs Begin with the Basics," *Computer Design.* August, 1983.

7. Reliability Analysis Center, *Reliability Design Handbook.* Chicago: ITT Research Institute, 1975.

5

The Feasibility Phase

New product ideas are not simply born. Companies in the medical device industry must study the marketplace. New product ideas come from examining the needs of hospitals, biomedical engineers, nurses, respiratory therapists physicians and other medical professionals as well as sales and marketing personnel. Many problems generally represent product opportunities.

The process of transforming product ideas into approved product development efforts begins with the definition of the customer's needs, the market and the intended application. This phase of development is characterized by several activities that must be successfully completed before proceeding to the design phase:

> Customer Survey
> Product Specification
> Reliability Goal
> Specification Review.

Each is a prerequisite for the succeeding one.

5.1 Customer Survey

The customer survey is an important tool in changing an idea into a product. The criticality of the survey is exhibited by an estimate that, on the average, it takes 58 initial ideas to get one commercially successful new product to market. It is therefore necessary to talk with various leaders in applicable markets to build a credible database of product ideas.

The market for a medical device is determined by the intended use of the device. Thus an electrocardiogram device has an applicable market in anesthesia, family practice, clinical testing and emergency rooms, to name a few. Some products, such as anesthesia vaporizers, have a more limited market potential.

Numerous methods of obtaining new product information exist including internal sources, industry leaders and technology analysis. Leaders in a particular field include medical practitioners and current or potential customers, who have published articles about a similar medical device or about potential applications in the particular field. Internal sources include a history of similar products, including history of failure and cost impact.

The survey consists of gathering information relative to the needs of the community, suggestions for improved methods of performing a task and ways to solve current problems. This data is screened and a business analysis conducted. The survey includes certain key questions:

> Where is the market now?
> Where will it go?
> How big is the potential market?
> What does the customer really want?
> How feasible is technical development?
> What are the chances of success?

The goal of the customer survey is to match the needs of the customer with the product concept.

5.2 Product Specification

The product specification is the first step in the process of transforming product ideas into approved product development efforts. This document is the result of the customer survey and subsequent interface between the Marketing, Design Engineering, Reliability Assurance and Regulatory Affairs personnel as it specifies what the product will do, how it will do it and how reliable it will be. To be effective, it must be as precise as possible.

The product specification should be a controlled document, that is, subject to revision level control, so that any changes that arise must be subjected in writing to the review process and approved prior to implementation. It prevents making verbal changes to the specification, without all concerned personnel informed. This will lead to confusion in later stages of development if the current specification is only a figment of someone's imagination or a pile of handwritten papers in someone's desk.

The specification should also have joint ownership. It should be written only after all concerned departments have discussed the concept and its alternatives and have agreed on the feasibility of the design. Agreement should come from Marketing, Design Engineering, Manufacturing, Customer Service, Reliability Assurance, Regulatory Affairs and Quality Assurance.

The specification is a detailed summary of the proposed product and includes:

> The type of product
> The market it addresses
> The function of the product
> The product parameters necessary to function effectively
> Accuracy requirements
> Tolerances necessary for function
> The anticipated environment for the device
> Cautions for aniticipated misuse
> Safety issues
> Human factors issues
> The anticipated life of the product
> The reliability goal
> Requirements from applicable domestic or international standards.

The parameter of particular interest to the Reliability Engineer is the reliability goal, which drives all subsequent activity.

5.3 Reliability Goal

The reliability goal is a statement of how effective the product is expected to be. The reliability goal is based upon several parameters:

> The anticipated life of the device
> The anticipated usage time per year
> The complexity of the device
> The anticipated use of the device
> The technology to be used
> The failure history of similar products.

The reliability goal may be defined in any of three ways:

> Reliability over a period of time
> Mean Time Between Failure
> Warranty cost as a percentage of sales.

The reliability goal may be specified as the desired reliability of the device over a specified period of time, i.e., the percentage of units still operational after the stated time period. For example, the reliability goal may state that the device must have a reliability of 0.99998 for an operational period of one year. This would mean 99.998% of the active units in the field would not have failed within one year.

The goal may be stated as a certain Mean Time Between Failure (MTBF). For example, the goal may be stated that a MTBF of 23,000 hours is desired. This would mean that 63% of the active units in the field would have failed once after 23,000 hours of operation.

The third method of stating the reliability goal is warranty cost. This is defined as the expenses a company incurs in order to guarantee their product will operate without failure for a certain amount of time, usually one year. It ordinarily includes:

> The cost of replaced or repaired parts
> The cost of Service's labor
> The cost of Service's travel.

Warranty cost directly reduces the profit from the device and may be an indicator of customer dissatisfaction. Warranty cost is typically stated as a percentage of sales.

Lower warranty cost means a more reliable device. It has been an industry standard for many years that a very successful company keeps its warranty cost at 3% of sales or less and a successful company keeps its warranty cost between 3% and 5% of sales. When the warranty cost rises above 5%, immediate action should be taken to bring it back within range, as the product expense will seriously affect profits.

The reliability goal may be determined by analyzing the cost impact of the product on the company's profit margin. The history of a similar device may be reviewed with special attention given to its failure pattern and the cost of those repairs.

For devices with no such history, the components may be analyzed for cost of repair or replacement and the ease of obtaining the parts. This will lead to a decision on the acceptable failure rate for the device.

Reliability, Mean Time Between Failure and Warranty can be calculated from each other. A detailed discussion of the mathematics involved can be found in the chapter on data analysis.

The reliability goal is a necessary parameter for the Reliability Engineer to plan subsequent activities. For example, when the MTBF and Reliability of the device is initially calculated from the parts list, the result will indicate whether the device will meet the reliability goal or whether the design must be revised. As various tests are conducted, results are related to either MTBF or Reliability. Again, this figure will be related to the reliablity goal to determine if the design meets the specification. Finally, as field data is collected and field MTBF and Reliability calculated, it ideally can be shown how the reliability has grown over time from the initial goal and has now surpassed it.

It would be simple to state the reliability goal as a Reliability of 1.0 or a MTBF of 1,000,000 hours or a warranty cost of 0%. This is an ideal situation, but practically impossible. Medical devices are designed, manufactured and serviced by human beings and therefore, at some time, may fail. It is the responsibility of development personnel to minimize the number and reduce the effects of such failures. Thus, the reliability goal should be a practical number based on a realistic set of parameters and any history of similar types of products. Unrealistic goals result in frustration and in unnecessary activities in an attempt to accomplish the impossible. It takes research and a realistic approach to the product to develop a reliability goal that everyone can live with.

5.4 Specification Review

Once the marketing survey is complete, the reliability goal established and the product specification drafted, a review of the draft is held. The review is attended by Managers from Marketing, Design Engineering, Manufacturing, Customer Service, Reliability Assurance, Regulatory Affairs, Safety and Quality Assurance. The draft of the specification is reviewed in detail. Discussion and appropriate action items are documented. Once the specification is approved, it is placed under revision level control. The review personnel establish the product development team, those personnel from each department who will be involved in the development process. The Product Manager is usually appointed from the Marketing department and the Product Development Manager is appointed from the Design Engineering department.

5.5 Summary

The Feasibility phase is the cornerstone of the Product Development Process. All activity depends on the requirements established from discussions with physicians and other medical personnel. These requirements are then formalized in a Product Specification, that not only details the technical requirements of the device, but the reliability goal as well. With the successful completion of the review, the development process moves into the design phase.

5.6 References

1. Lloyd, D. K. and M. Lipow, *Reliability Management, Methods and Mathematics*. 2nd Edition, Milwaukee, Wisconsin: The American Society for Quality Control, 1984.

2. Taylor, J. W. *Planning Profitable New Product Strategies*. Radnor, Pennsylvania: Chilton Book Company, 1984.

6

The Design Phase – The Device

Once the Product Specification is complete, the development process moves into the Design Phase. In this phase, the overall design and architecture of the device is conceived and made a reality. This phase is characterized by several activities general to the device, followed by parallel activities in hardware and software. The end of the design phase brings the hardware and software together. This chapter discusses the general activities, while the next two chapters discuss the hardware and software design activities separately.

6.1 System Specification

The first activity in the design phase is the creation of the System Specification from the previously approved Product Specification. The System Specification is created by the Design Engineering team as the approach to be taken in satisfying the design requirements.

The System Specification is a detailed description of how the design will be approached, the technology to be used, the functions that will be hardware-controlled and those that will be software-controlled. It addresses regulatory and standards issues, anticipated hazards which must be avoided, required system tolerances such as current or voltage and component tolerances such as resistor precision.

6.1.1 Hardware/Software Compatibility

An important area addressed in the System Specification is hardware/software compatibility. Often, during the product development process, hardware and software functions are being independently developed by separate groups of engineers. The groups will continue to work independently until someone realizes their products must function as a unit. It is very important to specify the hardware/software interface early in the design phase so that each group is aware of the other's activities and requirements.

The need for a reliable hardware/software interface has increased in importance due, in part, to increasing software-induced hardware failures that endanger system operations. Because hardware and software are different in nature, it is very difficult, if not impossible, to study the different types of failures and draw valid inferences by looking at the two systems separately. The two must be designed as a system.

The compatibility issue is specified according to:

> Hardware input
> Software input
> Interaction requirements
> System output
> Tolerances, if any.

6.2 Design Review

The System Specification is subjected to a design review attended by Design Engineering, Reliability Assurance, Quality Assurance, Regulatory Affairs, Manufacturing Engineering and Customer Service. The review is held prior to building any hardware or software modules, as concepts are more easily changed than actual hardware or code. The review addresses the design concept and its implication on reliability, manufacturing field service and standards/regulatory approvals.

Following the design review and subsequent changes to the System Specification, the specification becomes a controlled document. All changes to the specification would then be subject to an approval process prior to implementation.

6.3 Reliability Plan

The key to producing a successful product is to assure the device is reliable over its lifetime. To achieve this assurance, several essential activities must occur during the development process:

> Reliability must be designed into the device

> Reliability must be audited during development

> Cooperation between various development groups must be established.

The effort requires an organized approach to the Reliability Assurance activity. This organized approach is detailed in the Reliability Assurance Plan developed by the Reliability Assurance department in cooperation with Design Engineering and Marketing.

The Reliability Assurance Plan is a document detailing the Reliability Assurance activity to be conducted during the development process. The plan is product specific and addresses not only the general reliability issues associated with all devices, such as environmental testing or reliability demonstration, but also addresses the specific nuances of the individual device, such as anticipated hazards and specific pass/fail criteria for each test.

The document lists each anticipated reliability activity including:

> Test name
> Responsible department
> Test parameters
> Pass/fail criteria.

The document is reviewed and signed by Reliability Assurance, Design Engineering and Marketing. Sign-off indicates agreement on the process to be implemented and the desired results.

The Reliabilty Assurance Plan may included, but not be limited to the following activities, depending on the intended use and anticipated environment of the device:

> Documentation review
> Component/material qualification
> Reliability prediction
> Process evaluation
> Failure modes and effects analysis
> Use/misuse testing
> Environmental testing
> Electromagnetic compatibility testing
> Electrostatic discharge testing
> Simulated applications testing
> Reliability demonstration

6.4 Reliability Report

At the completion of the activity listed in the Reliability Assurance plan, a summary report is written listing the results of the activity. The report includes:

> Test conducted
> Test results
> Confidence level obtained

Analysis of failures
Mean Time Between Failure calculation
Redesign activities resulting from testing

The report also indicates whether the reliabiity goal was achieved or not.

Those activities listed in the Reliability Assurance Plan that were not performed or completed during the development process must be listed in the report as not being accomplished along with the justification for not performing or completing the activity.

6.5 Summary

A structured approach to the design of a medical device necessitates a layout of the design. The Engineering System Specification accomplishes this requirement. It forces the engineers to think through the design and how they plan to meet the device requirments. The time spent in thinking through the design shortens the "hands-on" design time.

Planning the reliability activity assists the Reliability Assurance personnel in assuring all areas of concern are addressed and that all test and standards requirments are accomplished.

6.6 References

1. Lloyd, D. K. and M. Lipow, *Reliability Management, Methods and Mathematics.* 2nd Edition Milwaukee, Wisconsin: The American Society for Quality Control, 1984.

2. Howell, J. M., "A Software Evaluation: Results and Recommendations," *Proceedings of the Reliability and Maintainability Symposium.* New York: Institute of Electrical and Electronic Engineers, 1983.

3. MIL-HDBK-217, *Reliability Prediction of Electronic Equipment.* Washington, DC: Department of Defense, 1986.

4. Romeu, J. L. and K. A. Dey, "Classifying Combined Hardware/Software Reliability Models," *Proceedings of the Annual Reliability and Maintainability Symposium.* New York: Institute of Electrical and Electronic Engineers, 1984.

7

The Design Phase – Hardware

Once the documentation describing the design and the organized approach to the design is complete, the actual design work begins. As the design activity proceeds, there are several failure-free or failure tolerant principles that must be considered to make the design more reliable, including:

Safety
Block diagram
Redundancy
Component selection
Component classification
Component derating
Safety margin
Load protection
Environmental conditions
Product misuse.

7.1 Safety

All medical devices must be safe, effective and reliable for their intended use. Safety must always be the most important design consideration. A device must never function or malfunction in a way that will cause harm to either the user or the patient. Safety is not an option, nor can it be attained solely through standards compliance.

Definitions of safety may vary, but the standard judicial test, under the theory of negligence, is whether or not the device is one that the ordinary, prudent firm would design, build and sell. The test, under the theories of strict liability and warranty, is whether the device itself is free of defects and not unreasonably dangerous for its intended and foreseeable use.

Mere compliance with applicable standards is not enough to assure a safe and effective device. Standards tend to lag the "state of art" by three to five years. Furthermore, standards are a one-way street in a lawsuit. Proof of compliance usually does little for a firm's defense; however, proof of noncompliance with standards often serves as a basis for punitive damages. Firms that are successful in the marketplace and the courtroom, however, are the ones that intentionally exceed safety and performance standards in their quest for safe, effective and reliable devices.

Figure 7.1 Block Diagram

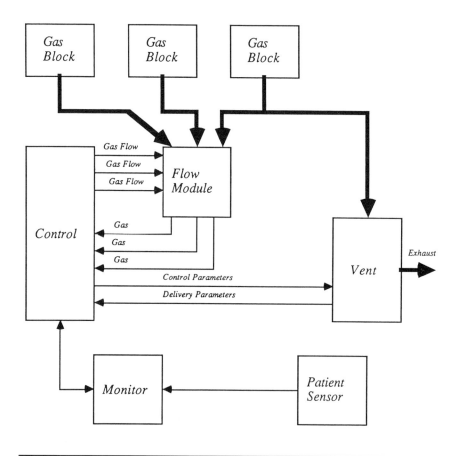

When designing for safety, there are two aspects to consider. The first is risk assessment that addresses the questions: What failure could cause harm to the patient or user? What misuse of the device could cause harm? These failures must be analyzed using such methods as fault tree analysis or failure mode analysis and must be designed out of the device.

The second aspect of safety is liability assessment. This addresses the questions: Have all possible failure modes been explored and designed out? Have all possible misuse situations been designed out or around? Court cases have special punitive judgements for companies that have knowledge about an unsafe condition and do nothing about it. Therefore, these areas must be analyzed and addressed.

7.2 Block Diagram

The first step in an organized design is the development of a block diagram of the device (see Figure 7.1). The block diagram is basically a flow chart of the signal movement within the device and is an aid to organizing the design. Individual blocks within the block diagram can be approached for component design, making the task more organized and less tedious. Once all blocks have been designed, their connections are all that remain.

7.3 Redundancy

One method of addressing the high failure rate of certain components is the use of redundancy, that is, the use of more than one component for the same purpose in the circuit. The philosophy behind redundancy is if one component fails, another will take its place and the operation will continue. An example would be the inclusion of two reed switches in parallel; if one fails because the reeds have stuck together, the other is available to continue the operation.

Redundancy may be of two types: active and standby.

7.3.1 Active Redundancy

Active redundancy occurs when two or more components are placed in parallel, with all components being operational. Satisfactory operation occurs if at least one of the components functions. If one component fails, the remaining parts function to sustain the operation.

Active redundancy is important in improving the reliability of a device. Placing components redundantly increases the Mean Time Between Failure (MTBF) of the circuit, thus improving reliability. Let's look at an example.

Figure 7.2 Circuit Example

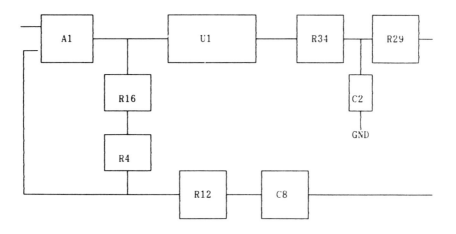

Figure 7.2 shows a circuit for an amplifier. Component U1 will be used as a candidate for redundancy. MIL-HDBK-217 gives a failure rate for the intended use of the component of 0.320 failures/million hours.

The failure rate assumption is that the component was in its useful life period. Therefore, the reciprocal of the failure rate is the MTBF.

When calculating the MTBF, the failure rate must be specified in failures per hour. Therefore, the failure rate, as listed in the handbook or in vendor literature must be divided by one million.

$$MTBF = 1/\lambda$$

$$= 1/0.00000032$$

$$= 3,125,000 \text{ hours}$$

Assume for a particular application, this MTBF value is not acceptable. One solution is to put two components in parallel (Figure 7.3).

Figure 7.3 Active Redundancy

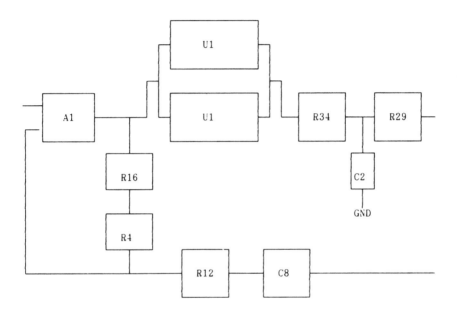

Again, it is assumed that the component is in its useful life period. For this case:

$$MTBF = 3/2\lambda$$
$$= 3/2(0.00000032)$$
$$= 3/0.00000064$$
$$= 4,687,500 \text{ hours}$$

By putting two components in active redundancy, the MTBF of the circuit has increased by 50% over the circuit containing one component.

7.3.2 Standby Redundancy

Standby redundancy occurs when two or more components are placed in parallel, but only one component is active. The remaining components remain in standby mode until activated.

Returning to the previous example, assume it has been decided to use standby redundancy to increase the reliability (Figure 7.4).

Again assuming the useful life period and ignoring the failure rate of the switch,

$$\text{MTBF} = 2/\lambda$$

$$= 2/0.00000032$$

$$= 6,250,000 \text{ hours}$$

By using standby redundancy, the MTBF has increased by 100% over the use of the single component and by 33% over active redundancy.

The use of redundancy at all is dependent upon the intended use of the circuit and the failure rates and cost of the individual components in the circuit. However, the use of redundancy definitely increases the reliability of the circuit. What type of redundancy is used again depends on the individual circuit and its intended application.

7.4 Component Selection

As certain portions of the design are finalized, the job of selecting the proper components for the design becomes a primary concern. In choosing components, one concern is long lead times for orders. Another relates to how vendors for these components are chosen. In many cases the three main criteria for choosing a component vendor are:

1. Lowest cost
2. Lowest cost
3. Lowest cost.

Loyalty to a particular vendor may also be a practical consideration. If the design is to be reliable, however, the component parameters of choice include:

Fitness for use
Criticality vs non-criticality
Reliability
History
Safety.

7.4.1 Component Fitness for Use

Fitness for use includes analyzing a component for the purpose to which it is designed. Many vendors list common applications for their components and tolerances for those applications. Where the desired applica-

Figure 7.4 Standby Redundancy

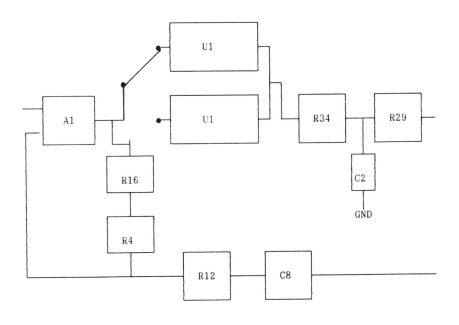

tion is different from that listed, the component must be analyzed and verified in that application. This includes specifying parameters particular to its intended use, specifying tolerances, inclusion of a safety margin and a review of the history of the part in other applications.

For components being used for the first time in a particular application and for which no history or vendor data is available, testing in the desired application should be conducted. More is said about this in the chapter on validation.

7.4.2 Component Criticality

The term "critical" is one of the most misused terms when discussing component and device usage. The term "critical" has an explicitly defined meaning for medical devices and should not be used in other situations. As listed in FDA documents and other standards, two definitions are significant.

A critical device is any device that is intended for surgical implant into the body or to support or sustain life, and whose failure to perform, when properly used, in accordance with instructions for use, provided in the labeling, can be reasonably expected to result in a significant injury to the user It is any device so identified as "critical" by the FDA or any other national regulatory agency. Current critical devices listed by the FDA, include:

> Anesthesia machines
> Blood Pumps
> Breathing Circuits
> Defibrillators
> Hemodialysis Systems
> Incubators
> Oxygenators
> Pacemakers
> Infusion Pumps
> Neural Stimulators
> Replacement Heart Valves
> Ventilators.

A critical component is any component of a critical device whose failure to perform can reasonably be expected to cause the safety and effectiveness of a device to be altered in such a manner as to result in significant user injury, death or a clearly diminished capacity to function as an otherwise normal human being.

These two definitions contain two very important ideas.

> A critical component can only exist in a critical device

> A critical device does not necessarily contain a critical component.

If the device is not listed as critical by the FDA or other regulatory agency, there is no critical component. It may be significant for an application, but is not "critical."

If the device is listed as critical, each component must be analyzed for its application and the effect of a single point failure. From this information, decide which, if any of the components, are critical. This analysis should be based on the functionality of the device, the functionality of the component, the effectiveness of maintaining high reliability in the component and traceability considerations.

FDA regulations contain certain requirements for all critical components:

> Written procedures for acceptance, sampling and testing
> Inspection sample size based on statistical rationale
> Each lot identified with a control number
> The percentage of defective parts recorded
> Vendor agreement to notify the manufacturer of design changes
> Traceability.

The critical components of a critical device should be chosen by the product development team based on their function within the device. Design Engineering and Reliability Assurance should review all components in the device to determine which meet the definition of criticality.

7.4.3 Component Reliability

The process of assuring the reliability of a component is a multi-step procedure, including:

> Initial vendor assessment
> Vendor audit
> Vendor evaluation
> Vendor qualification.

The initial vendor assessment should be a review of any past history of parts delivery, including on time deliveries, incoming rejection rate, willingness of the vendor to work with the company and handling of rejected components. The vendor should be questioned as to the nature of his acceptance criteria, what type of reliability tests are performed and what the results of the tests are. It is also important to determine whether the nature of the test performed is relevant to the application and the environment the component will experience in the device. A checklist is an aid during the assessment (Figure 7.5).

Once the initial vendor assessment is satisfactorily completed, an audit of the vendor's facility is in order. The vendor's processes should be reviewed, the production capabilities assessed, rejection rates and failure analysis discussed. Sometimes the appearance of the facility provides a clue as to the type of vendor. A facility that is unorganized or dirty, for example, suggests a poor quality of work performed.

Once components are shipped, it is desirable that the quality of the incoming product is what is expected. A typical approach to the evalua-

Figure 7.5 Sample Vendor Assessment Checklist

```
                    Vendor Audit Checklist

     Vendor_____     Date_____
```

	Yes	No*
1. The vendor maintains a Quality Assurance Manual.		
2. The vendor's purchase orders clearly specify acceptance criteria.		
3. Receiving inspection records reflect a quality history.		
4. The vendor uses a positive means of identification of all stock.		
5. The vendor operates a system that assures uninspected parts will not be used.		
6. The vendor maintains a system for the proper identification of the inspection status of in-process materials.		
7. The vendor maintains a system for periodically calibrating tools and gauges.		
8. The vendor maintains written procedures for calibrating measuring devices.		
9. The vendor maintains standard operating procedures in the manufacturing area.		
10. Drawings used in manufacturing and test are legible and reflect the latest changes.		
11. The vendor maintains a program for analyzing failed components and assemblies.		
13. Reports on nonconforming materials are regularly prepared and are reviewed by management for action.		

```
     *Use this space for explanation when "No" is indicated
```

tion would be to do 100% inspection on the first several lots to check for consistent quality. Once the quality of the incoming material has been obtained and it is consistently satisfactory, components can be randomly inspected or inspected on a skip-lot basis.

Many companies have established a system of qualified vendors to determine what components will be used and the extent of incoming inspection. Some vendors qualify through a rigorous testing scheme that determines the incoming components meet the specification. Other companies have based qualification on a certain number of deliveries with no failures at incoming. Only components from qualified vendors should be used in any medical device. This is especially important when dealing with critical components.

7.4.4 Component History
Component history is an important tool in deciding what components to use in a design. It is important to review the use of the component in previous products including the incoming rejection history, performance of the component in field use and failure rate history.

A helpful tool in looking at component history is the use of available data banks of component information. One such data bank is MIL-HDBK-217. This military standard lists component failure rates based upon the environment in which they are used. The information has been accumulated from the use of military hardware. Some environments are similar to that seen by medical devices and the data is applicable. MIL-HDBK-217 is discussed in greater detail later in this chapter.

Another good source of component data is a government program named GIDEP (Government-Industry Data Exchange Program). To join the program you must submit a report listing failure rates of components in your particular applications. You then receive reports listing summaries of other reports the group has received. It is a good way to get a history on components you intend to use. More information may be obtained by writing to:

> GIDEP Operations Center
> Department of the Navy
> Naval Weapons Station
> Seal Beach, Corona Annex
> Corona, CA 91720, USA

7.4.5 Component Safety
The safety of each component in the application must be analyzed. This is done by performing a fault tree analysis, where possible failures are

traced back to the components causing them.

Fault tree analysis is a stepwise sequential process beginning with the collection of appropriate documentation for creating the fault tree. This documentation includes parts lists, operating environment requirements and user manual. Once the documentation is reviewed, a failure is chosen that becomes the top event on the tree. This failure should be well defined and measurable. Branches from the top event are drawn to the events on the next level that could cause the top event. The secondary events are then analyzed to determine their causes. This continues until the lowest level is composed of basic fault events. The tree is repeated for each failure to be analyzed. The details of developing a fault tree are discussed in section 9.3.4.1.

A failure mode analysis is essential in reviewing single point failures of components. Unlike the fault tree, which works from the failure back to the component, failure mode analysis works from the component to the resultant failure.

Failure modes and effects analysis is a test conducted to determine the effect of a single point failure on the output of a device. The test may be performed on a breadboard or PC boards where integrated circuits are socketed. Components are subjected to certain failure modes while monitoring the output of the device. The effect of the failure mode is recorded and analyzed for safety concerns. The details of the failure modes and effects analysis are discussed in section 9.3.5.

7.5 Component Classification

One method of organizing components and determining future activity is to classify each component in its intended application in one of three mutually exclusive categories. The evaluation criteria include:

> Safety
> Product Function
> Parts Cost.

Each component should be classified as to its potential safety hazard if it fails. The component must be analyzed in its particular application because a component failure may present a safety hazard in one application and no safety hazard in another.

Each component should be classified as to the effect on the systems operation if it fails. Thus a component failure may render the device inoperative, it may have the potential for rendering the device inoperative or it may not render the device inoperative, but may be an inconvenience for the customer.

Components may also be classified according to their cost. Thus it may be cost effective to burn-in an expensive component in order to reduce the number of infant mortality failures, thus saving the cost of replacement.

Figure 7.6 illustrates one example of a component classification system. From this chart, one could determine component burn-in activities. For example, Class I parts would require burn-in prior to use. Class II parts would have their burn-in status determined by the product development team, based upon the application. Class III parts would not require a burn-in. Component burn-in will be discussed in more detail in the chapter on Manufacturing.

As an example of the classification, consider an IC used in an anesthesia ventilator. If the integrated circuit fails and causes the ventilator to cease functioning, the integrated circuit would be considered Level I because its failure would cause a safety hazard to the patient. The safety concern is the reason for Level I.

If the same integrated circuit were used in a blood pressure monitor and its failure caused the monitor to cease operation, the integrated circuit would be considered Level II. In this case there is not safety hazard to the patient, but the system is rendered inoperable.

If the same integrated circuit is used in a digital thermometer and its failure caused the digital display to blink, the integrated circuit would be considered Level III. Here there is no safety hazard nor is the system rendered inoperative. The blinking display is hard to read and therefore is an inconvenience to the user.

The classification by cost is important when a component is expensive and replacement would be costly. In this case burn-in is an acceptable means to reduce the failure rate.

7.6 Component Derating

Component failure in a given application is determined by the interaction between the strength and the stress level. As the operational stress levels of a component exceed the rated strength of the component, the failure rate increases. As the operational stress level fall below the rated strength, the failure rate decreases.

Component derating is the use of components at considerably lowers than rated stress levels, for example, the use of a 2 watt resistor in a 1 watt application. It has been shown that derating a component to 50% of its operating value generally decreases its failure rate by a factor greater than 30%. As the failure rate is decreased, the reliability is increased.

Components are derated with respect to those stresses to which the component is most sensitive. These stresses fall into two categories, operational stresses and application stresses. These include:

Operational	Application
Temperature	Voltage
Humidity	Current
Atmospheric Pressure	Friction
	Vibration

7.7 Safety Margin

Components or assemblies will fail when the applied load exceeds the strength at the time of application. The consideration of the load should take into account combined loads, such as voltage and temperature or

Figure 7.6 Component Classification Chart

Level	Safety Concern	Operational Concern	Cost Concern
I	Failure results in a potential safety hazard	Failure renders the system inoperative	Not applicable
II	Failure results in no safety hazard	Failure results in the potential for rendering the system inoperative	$5.00 or greater
III	Failure results in no safety hazard	Failure may cause customer inconvenience	Less than $5.00

humidity and friction. Combined loads can have effects which are out of proportion to their separate contributions, both in terms of instantaneous effects and strength degradation effects.

Determining the acceptable tolerance ranges for component parameters is an essential element of assuring adequate safety margins. Tolerancing, with appropriate controls on manufacturing provides control over the resulting strength distributions. Analysis should be based on worst case strength or distributional analysis, rather than on an anticipated strength distribution.

Safety margin is calculated as follows:

Safety Margin = (Mean safety factor) - 1

= (Mean strength/mean stress) - 1

An example illustrates the concept:

A structure is required to withstand a pressure of 20,000 psi. A safety margin of 0.5 is to be designed into the device. What is the strength that must be designed in?

Safety Margin = (strength/stress) - 1

0.5 = (strength/20,000) - 1

1.5 = strength/20,000

(20,000 x 1.5) = strength

30,000 psi = strength

Most handbooks list a safety margin of 2.0 as the minimum required for high reliability devices. In some cases, this may result in an overdesign. The safety margin must be evaluated according to device function, the importance of its application and the safety requirements. For most medical applications, a minimum safety margin of 0.5 is adequate.

7.8 Load Protection

Protection against extreme loads should be considered whenever practicable. In many cases, extreme loading situations can occur and must be protected against. When overload protection is provided, the reliability analysis should be performed on the basis of the maximum load which can be anticipated, bearing in mind the tolerances of the protection system.

7.9 Environmental Protection

Medical devices should be designed to withstand the worst case environmental conditions in the product specification, with a safety margin included. Typical environmental ranges which a device may experience have been defined by various standard organizations in the United States and overseas. European standards contain the worst case ranges, including:

Operating temperature	0 to +55 degrees centigrade
Storage temperature	−40 to +65 degrees centigrade
Humidity	95% RH at 40 degrees centigrade
Mechanical vibration	5 to 300 Hz at 2 Gs
Mechanical shock	24″ to 48″ drop
Mechanical impact	10 Gs at a 50 msec pulse width
Electrostatic discharge	Up to 50,000 volts

Electromagnetic compatibility becomes an issue in an environment like an operating room. Each medical device should be protected from interference from other equipment, such as electrocautery and should be designed to eliminate radiation to other equipment.

7.10 Product Misuse

An area of design concern that was briefly addressed earlier in this chapter is the subject of product misuse. Whether through failure to properly read the operation manual or through improper training, medical devices are going to be misused and even abused. There are many stories of product misuse, such as the hand held monitor that was dropped into the toilet bowl, the user who used a hammer to pound a 9 volt battery into a monitor backwards or the user who spilled a can of soda on and into a device. Practically, it is impossible to make a device completely misuse-proof. But it is highly desirable to design around the ones that can be anticipated.

Some common examples of product misuse include:

Excess application of cleaning solutions
Physical abuse
Spills
Excess weight applied to certain parts
Excess torque applied to controls or screws

> Improper voltages, frequencies or pressures
> Improper or interchangeable electrical or
> pneumatic connections

Product misuse should be discussed with Marketing to define as many possible misuse situations as can be anticipated. The designer must then design around these situations, including a safety margin, which will serve to increase the reliability of the device. Where design restrictions limit the degree of protection against misuse and abuse, the device should alarm or should malfunction in a manner that is harmless and obvious to the user.

7.11 Initial Reliability Prediction

Once the design has proceeded to the point where parts have been defined and a parts list developed, an initial prediction based on the parts used may be performed to produce an initial MTBF value. This value may then be compared to the original reliability goal to determine if the design will meet it. The initial prediction is also used to highlight certain areas of the design that have a high failure rate, such as a particular component or an assembly, (e.g., a PC board or a pneumatic circuit.) The prediction forms the basis for future analysis, reliability growth and change.

Certain limitations exist with the prediction method. The first deals with the ability to accumulate data of known validity for the new application. The design may contain many new components, some of which are new to the marketplace and are not included in MIL-HDBK-217. Also, a component may be used in an application for which failure rate data has not been accumulated. In these cases, vendor data must be obtained or the history of similar components in similar products must be obtained to complete the prediction.

A second limitation is the complexity of the predicting technique. It takes a long time to list each component, look up each failure rate and then calculate the MTBF for each assembly and then the device. As the complexity of the product increases, the length of time increases. Several companies have advertised computer programs that perform the prediction. The program takes the individual components and their quantity and determines the failure rates from tables residing in the computer, which are periodically updated.

MIL-HDBK-217 contains two methods of doing a prediction, a parts stress analysis and a part count analysis. The parts stress analysis requires a greater amount of detail to complete, is applicable at a later stage in development when hardware testing has been completed. The parts count analysis requires minimum information - the identities and quantities of parts, quality levels and application environment. Because it does not require operational stress levels, it can be performed early in the design phase as soon as a parts list is developed. Only the parts count method will be discussed here. Details of the parts stress analysis may be found in MIL-HDBK-217.

7.11.1 Parts Count Prediction

There are four items necessary to begin a parts count prediction:

> A schematic
> A parts list
> MIL-HDBK-217
> Marketing parameters.

The marketing parameters include 1) the use rate, i.e., the number of hours the device is in operation per day, the number of days per week and the number of weeks per year, 2) the desired MTBF goal, 3) the desired life of the device and 4) the desired warranty cost as a percentage of sales. These parameters are used for final calculations after the MTBF has been calculated.

The first step in completing a part count prediction is to choose the environment in which the product will be used from among the many listed in the handbook. The three most commonly experienced by medical devices, in order of increasing severity, are:

> GF   Ground Fixed
>
> Conditions less than ideal, such as installation in permanent racks, with adequate cooling air and possible installation in unheated buildings.
>
> An example would be a wall-mounted gas pressure alarm.
>
> GB   Ground Benign
>
> Nonmobile, laboratory environment, readily accessible to maintenance.
>
> An example would be CAT scan residing in one location or a monitor permanently set on a table or desk.

GM   Ground Mobile

Equipment installed on wheeled or tracked vehicles.

An example would be an evoked potential system that can be rolled from the operating room into a patient's room or a laboratory.

Where a question exists as to which of two environments should be chosen, select the more severe of the two.

Once the environment is identified, all parts in one particular assembly, such as a PC board or a pnuematic circuit, are listed on a form, such as that shown in Figure 7.7. The form lists the type of component, the style of part where applicable, the quantity of that component in the assembly, the failure rate for that component, and the total failure rate for the quantity of that component.

When all parts are listed on the sheet, start the process of determining the individual failure rates. The individual components are found in the appropriate tables within the parts count analysis portion of MIL-HDBK-217. The base failure rate is listed as well as the quality factor and other parameters, where necessary. The component failure rate is found by multiplying the base failure rate and the quality factor and other listed factors. This number is then listed in the individual component failure rate. This number is multiplied by the quantity included in the assembly and the total failure rate is determined. This process continues for the remainder of the items in the assembly. When all components are determined, the total failure rates are summed to determine the failure rate for the assembly. This failure rate is listed as failure per million hours. To calculate the MTBF for the assembly, the total failure rate is divided by one million and the reciprocal taken. This will be the MTBF in hours.

The above process is repeated for each assembly. When completed, the total failure rates for each assembly are summed, yielding the total failure rate for the device (Figure 7.8). The MTBF for the device is calculated as it was above, for the assembly.

An example illustrates the application method.

7.11.2 Parts Count Prediction Example

A company is developing the Model 3322 Monitor. It is a device consisting of a computer system, Winchester, printer, and two additional boards. The Reliability Assurance department has been given the task of determining the MTBF and warranty cost for the unit based on hardware components used.

Figure 7.7 Parts Count Prediction Sheet

INITIAL RELIABILITY PREDICTION

Device_____

Assembly_____ Date_____

Component	Style	Quanitity	Individual Failure Rate	Total Failure Rate

Total Failure Rate   _____

MTBF   _____

The device will be stationary during use. Thus the environment "GB" is chosen. The parts for each board are listed on separate worksheets and the failure rates calculated. Figure 7.9 shows a sample worksheet for the ADC board.

The PC board is listed in Table 5.2-30 (Figure 7.10) under the term 'PC Bs.' Read across the line until the column GB is found. The value there is 0.0027. The Quality Factor for the interconnects is found in Table 5.2-31 (Figure 7.11). Since this board is a MIL-SPEC board, the quality factor is 1. Therefore, the failure rate for the board is 0.0027 failures per million hours.

The resistors used are type "RN." The data for resistors are found in Table 5.2-27 (Figure 7.12). Find Style "RN" and the column GB. The value is 0.007. The quality value for resistors of two letter types, found in Table 5.2-29 (Figure 7.13), is 1. Therefore, the failure rate for the resistors is 0.007.

To find integrated circuit data, for example 54LS164, the cross reference table 5.1.2.7-17 (Figure 7.14), is used. Locate 54LS164 in the table. It references the number 30605 in table 5.1.2.7-18 (Figure 7.15). That table lists the complexity for 30605 as 36 gates. Then turning to table 5.2-2 (Figure 7.16), under MOS for 1 to 100 gates, look under the column marked GB and find the value 0.009. Since the integrated circuit is to be burned-in, quality level B-2 is used. Table 5.2.23 (Figure 7.17) lists the quality level as 5. The quality level is multiplied by the failure rate, giving a total failure rate of 0.045 failures per million hours.

Other parts have their failure rates calculated in the same manner, using the appropriate handbook tables. Figure 7.9 is a list of those failure rates, summed to give the total failure rate for the board. The failure rate is then divided by one million and the reciprocal taken, to give the MTBF in hours.

The total failure for the device is calculated by summing the individual failure rates for the components (Figure 7.18). The parts previously calculated are included along with other components whose failure rate was obtained by getting the vendor's data. Thus, the manufacturer of the printer, after conducting tests, calculated a failure rate of 17.544 failures per million hours, or a MTBF of 57,000 hours. The total device failure rate is 114.275 failures per million hours or a MTBF of 8751 hours. This indicates 63% of the active units will have experienced one failure within the first 8751 hours of operation.

The next task is to calculate the warranty cost for the device. To do this, several parameters need to be known. For this monitor, Marketing has determined the unit will operate 2500 hours per year (10 hours per

Figure 7.8 Device Prediction Sheet

INITIAL RELIABILITY PREDICTION
SUMMARY SHEET

Device_____

Date_____

Assembly	Quantity	Total Failure Rate

Device Failure Rate   ——————————————

Device MTBF   ——————————————

Figure 7.9 Sample Worksheet

INITIAL RELIABILITY PREDICTION

Device_____Model 3322 Monitor_____

Assembly_____ADC Board____   Date_5/3/89_____

Component	Style	Quantity	Individual Failure Rate	Total Failure Rate
PC Board		1	0.0027	0.0027
Resistors	RN	30	0.007	0.210
Capacitors	CK	5	0.004	0.020
Capacitors	CM	10	0.003	0.030
Diodes	Zener	18	0.022	0.396
Transistors	SI NPN	8	0.003	0.024
54LS164		2	0.045	0.090
8259		1	0.055	0.055
54LS240		3	0.045	0.155
54LS00		5	0.030	0.150

Total Failure Rate   1.133 fr/million hrs

MTBF   882,613 hours

Figure 7.10 Table 5.2-30

PART TYPE	USE ENVIRONMENT			
	ARW	AUT	CL	GB
SWITCHES				
Toggle & Push Button	0.046	0.01	1.2	0.001
Sensitive	6.9	1.5	180.0	0.15
Thumbwheel	26.0	5.6	670.0	0.56
Other Rotary	15.0	3.3	400.0	0.33
CIRCUIT BREAKERS				
Thermal	5.2	1.0	N/A	0.11
Magnetic	2.8	0.54	N/A	0.06
CONNECTORS				
Cir/Rack/Panel	0.56	0.34	5.1	0.0055
Coaxial	0.55	0.32	5.3	0.006
PCBs	0.096	0.14	2.6	0.0027
IC SOCKETS	0.048	0.019	1.3	0.0019
INTERCONNECT ASSY	0.78	0.62	21.0	0.041
TUBES	See section 5.1.4			
LASERS	See section 5.1.5			

day, 5 days per week, 50 weeks per year). Two hundred units will be sold the first year. The selling price per unit will be $58000. The average charge for a service call is $850.

$$\text{Total Sales} = 200 \text{ units } (\$58,000)$$
$$= \$11,600,000$$

Figure 7.11 Table 5.2-31

PART TYPE	QUALITY LEVEL	
	MIL-SPEC	NON-MIL
MAGNETRONS	N/A	N/A
INDUCTIVE	1	3
MOTORS	1	6
RELAYS, SOLID STATE	1	3
RELAYS, TIME DELAY	1	4
RELAYS, ALL OTHERS	1	6
SWITCHES, TOGGLE & SENSITIVE	1	20
SWITCHES, THUMBWHEEL	1	1.5
SWITCHES, OTHER ROTARY TYPES	1	50
CIRCUIT BREAKERS	1	8.4
CONNECTORS	1	3
INTERCONNECTION ASSEMBLIES	1	10

Figure 7.12 Table 5.2-27

RESISTORS, FIXED			USE ENVIRONMENT		
CONSTRUCTION	STYLE	MIL-SPEC	AUT	GMS	GB
Composition	RCR	39008	0.017	0.0006	0.0005
	RC	11	0.083	0.0030	0.0025
Film	RLR	39017	0.012	0.0015	0.0012
	RL	22684	0.060	0.0074	0.0062
	RNR	55182	0.014	0.0017	0.0014
	RN	10509	0.069	0.0083	0.0069
Film, power	RD	11804	0.210	0.0140	0.0120
Film, network	RZ	83401	0.630	0.0300	0.0250
Wirewound	RBR	39005	0.270	0.0100	0.0085
Accurate	RB	93	1.400	0.0510	0.0430
Wirewound	RWR	39007	0.150	0.0150	0.0140
Power	RW	26	0.760	0.0760	0.0690
Wirewound	RER	39009	0.094	0.0095	0.0080
Ch. Mount	RE	18546	0.470	0.0480	0.0400

Figure 7.13 Table 5.2-29

FAILURE RATE LEVEL	QUALITY FACTOR
L	1.5
M	1.0
P	0.3
R	0.1
S	0.03

For non-ER parts (styles with only 2 letters in
Tables 5.2-27 and 5.2-28), the quality factor = 1
providing parts are procured in accordance with the
part specification; if procured as commercial (NON-
MIL) quality, the quality factor = 3. For ER parts
(styles with 3 letters), use the quality factor
value for the "letter" failure rate level procured.

The reliability of the device based on the 2500 hour operating time per year is:

$$\text{Reliability} = \exp(\text{-use time/MTBF})$$

$$= \exp(\text{-2500/8751})$$

$$= \exp(\text{-0.2857})$$

$$= 0.75$$

This means 75% of the 200 units will survive the first year without a failure, while 25% or 50 units will fail.

The total Service charge is:

$$\text{Service charge} = 50 \text{ units (\$850)}$$

$$= \$42,500$$

The warranty cost as a percentage of sales is thus:

$$\text{Warranty Cost} = \$42,500/\$11,600,000$$

$$= 0.0037$$

$$= 0.37\% \text{ of sales}$$

Figure 7.14 Table 5.1.2.7-17

COMMERCIAL	M38510/	COMMERCIAL	M38510/	COMMERCIAL	M38510/
5409	01602	54116	01503	54F151	33901
54S09	08004	5412	00106	54153	01403
54LS09	31005	54LS12	30006	54S153	07902
5410	00103	54121	01201	54LS153	30902
54L10	02003	54L121	04201	54F153	33902
54H10	02303	54122	01202	54154	15201
54S10	07005	54L122	04202	54155	15202
54LS10	30005	54LS122	31403	54LS155	32601
54F10	33003	54123	01203	54156	15203
54ALS10	37002	54LS123	31401	54LS156	32602
54HC10	65002	54LS124	31701	54157	01405
54ALS1000	38401	54125	15301	54S157	07903
54ALS1002	38402	54LS125	32301	54LS157	30903
54ALS1003	38403	54LS125A	32301	54F157	33903
54ALS1004	38409	54126	15302	54S158	07904
54ALS1005	38410	54LS126	32302	54LS158	30904
54ALS1008	38404	5413	15101	54F158	33904
54H101	02205	54LS13	31301	5416	00802
54ALS1010	38405	54132	15103	54160	01303
54ALS1011	38406	54LS132	31303	54LS160	31503
54ALS1020	38407	54HC132	65005	54LS160A	31503
54H103	02206	54S133	07009	54161	01306
54ALS1032	38408	54ALS133	37005	54LS161	31504
54ALS1034	38411	54S134	07010	54LS161A	31504
54ALS1035	38412	54S135	07502	54162	01305
54107	00203	54S138	07701	54LS162	31511
54LS107	30108	54LS138	30701	54LS162A	31511
54LS109	30109	54ALS138	37701	54163	01304
54F109	34102	54S139	07702	54LS163	31512
54ALS109	37102	54LS139	30702	54LS163A	31512
54S11	08001	5414	15102	54164	00903
54H11	15502	54LS14	31302	54L164	02802
54LS11	31001	54S140	08101	54LS164	30605
54F11	34002	54145	01005	54165	00904
54ALS11	37402	54147	15601	54LS165	30608
54S112	07102	54148	15602	54LS165A	30608
54LS112	30103	54LS148	36001	54LS166	30609
54F112	34103	54S15	08002	54LS168	31505
54ALS112A	37103	54LS15	31002	54LS169	31506
54S113	07103	54150	01401	54LS169A	31506
54LS113	30104	54151	01406	5417	00804
54S114	07104	54S151	07901	54170	01801
54LS114	30105	54LS151	30901	54LS170	31902

Figure 7.15 Table 5.1.2.7-18

M38510/ XXXXXX	COMPLEXITY (# of gates)	Np	M38510/ XXXXXX	COMPLEXITY (# of gates)	Np
30502	4	14	30903	15	16
30601	47	16	30904	15	16
30602	41	16	30905	17	16
30603	37	14	30906	15	16
30604	39	16	30907	15	16
30605	36	14	30908	16	16
30606	48	14	30909	15	16
30607	48	16	31001	3	14
30608	62	16	31002	3	14
30609	68	16	31003	2	14
30701	16	16	31004	4	14
30702	18	16	31005	4	14
30703	18	16	31101	31	16
30704	44	16	31201	42	16
30801	63	24	31202	42	16
30901	17	16	31301	2	14
30902	16	16			

Some of the failure rates are estimates that may improve after reliability testing. Prior experience, comparing initial predictions with actual field data, has shown that the parts count predictions are usually on the pessimistic side by 10% to 20%. However, the predictions are good indicators of trends with regard to warranty costs, serve to highlight parts of the device that have high failure rates and provide valuable information for the Service organization, in planning the inventory of replacement parts for the device. Predictions can be updated, with greater confidence levels, when reliability testing is accomplished.

7.12 Design Reviews

Despite discipline, training and care, it is inevitable that occasional oversights or errors will occur in new designs. Design reviews are held to highlight critical aspects of the design and to focus attention on possible shortfalls.

Figure 7.16 Table 5.2.2

DEVICE DESCRIPTION		APPLICATION ENVIRONMENT		
NUMBER OF GATES	TECHNOLOGY	GB	GF	GM
1 - 100	BIPOLAR	0.0061	0.0222	0.0349
	MOS	0.0094	0.0323	0.0517
>100 - 1,000	BIPOLAR	0.0115	0.0391	0.0608
	MOS	0.0179	0.0593	0.0945
>1,000 - 3,000	BIPOLAR	0.0225	0.0750	0.1164
	MOS	0.0354	0.1155	0.1837
>3,000 - 10,000	BIPOLAR	0.0604	0.2519	0.4039
	MOS	0.0863	0.3330	0.5386
>10,000 - 30,000	BIPOLAR	0.1066	0.4103	0.6507
	MOS	0.1584	0.5724	0.9200

A design review is held to:

Review the progress of the design
Monitor reliability growth
Assure reliability requirements are being met
Provide information to all concerned with the project

The primary purpose of the design review is to make a choice among alternative design approaches. The output of this review should include an understanding of the weak areas in the chosen design and the areas in need of special attention in order to improve reliability. Areas which should be covered during the design review include:

Redundancy versus derating
Redesign of weak areas versus high reliability parts
Review product misuse

Figure 7.17 Table 5.2-23

QUALITY LEVEL	DESCRIPTION	QUALITY FACTOR
S	Procured in full accordance with MIL-M-38510, Class S requirements. Class S listing on QPL-38510.	0.25
S-1	Procured in full compliance with the requirements of MIL-STD-975 or MIL-STD-1547 and have procuring activity specification approval.	0.75
B	Procured in full accordance with MIL-M-38510, Class B requirements. Class B listing on QPL-38510.	1.0
B-1	Fully compliant with all requirements of paragraph 1.2.1 of MIL-STD-883 and procured to a MIL drawing, DESC drawing or other government approved document.	2.0
B-2	Not fully compliant with requirements of paragraph 1.2.1 of MIL-STD-883 and procured to government approved documentation including vendor's equivalent Class B requirements.	5.0
D	Hermetically sealed parts with normal reliability screening and manufacturer's quality assurance practices. Non hermetic parts encapsulated with organic material must be subjected to 160 hours burn-in at 125 degrees C, 10 temperature cycles (-55 C to 125 C) with end point electricals and high temperature continuity test at 100 degrees C.	10.0
D-1	Commercial or non-mil standard part, encapsulated or sealed with organic materials (e.g., epoxy, silicone or phenolic)	20.0

Figure 7.18 Device Total Failure Rate

INITIAL RELIABILITY PREDICTION

SUMMARY SHEET

Device___Model 3322 Monitor_____

Date__May 10, 1989_____

Assembly	Quantity	Total Failure Rate
Computer System	1	59.649
Winchester	1	25.000
Printer	1	17.544
ADC Board	1	1.133
Mother Board	1	10.949

Device Failure Rate   114.275 failures/million hours

Device MTBF   8751 hours

Review areas of overstress
Parts classification
Determine if all requirements of the specification have
been satisfied.

The design review should follow a structured order and be well documented, with decisions, action items and responsibilities listed. Some people believe checklists are helpful in design reviews. If used, they should contain questions pertinent to the particular application of the device.

7.13 Summary

Hardware validation is an important part of the Product Development Process. Components must be qualified for their intended use, parts of the device with the potential for high failure rates must be identified, tolerances and safety margins must be tested to assure they are adequate and anticipated misuse of the device must be checked to assure it will not cause a failure. In addition, the design must meet its reliability and financial goals and still be delivered on time.

The next chapter discusses the other major portion of design activity – software design.

7.14 References

1. Connors, T. J., "The Cost of Screening vs Not Screening," *Evaluation Engineering.* July/August, 1978.

2. Department of Health, Education and Welfare, *Device GMP: A Quality Audit Program for Industry.* Silver Spring, Maryland: Food and Drug Administration, 1979.

3. Government-Industry Data Exchange Program, *Program Summary.* June, 1979.

4. Jensen, F. and N. E. Peterson, *Burn-In.* New York: John Wiley and Sons, 1982.

5. Lloyd, D. K. and M. Lipow, *Reliability Management, Methods and Management.* 2nd Edition Milwaukee, Wisconsin: American Society for Quality Control, 1984.

6. MIL-STD-202, *Test Methods for Electronic and Electrical Component Parts.* Washington, DC: Department of Defense, 1980.

7. MIL-HDBK-217, *Reliability Prediction of Electronic Equipment.* Washington, DC: Department of Defense, 1986.

8. MIL-STD-750, *Test Methods for Semiconductor Devices.* Washington, DC: Department of Defense, 1983.

9. MIL-STD-781, *Reliability Design Qualification and Production Acceptance Tests: Exponential Distribution.* Washington, DC: Department of Defense, 1977.

10. MIL-STD-883, *Test Methods and Procedures for Microelectronics.* Washington, DC: Department of Defense, 1983.

11. O'Connor, P. D. T., *Practical Reliability Engineering.* New York: John Wiley and Sons, 1984.

12. Oppenheimer, C. D., "Reliable Designs Begin with the Basics," *Computer Design.* August, 1983.

8

The Design Phase – Software

A second major activity in the design of a medical device is software development. Like hardware, the software must be designed to enhance the safety, effectiveness and reliability of the device. Software cannot be dealt with in the same manner as hardware.

8.1 Hardware vs Software

Software differs from hardware in several respects:

Software components do not degrade; hardware components do

Software processes are not constrained by the laws of physics; hardware processes are

Software interfaces are conceptual as opposed to the physical interfaces of hardware

The failure modes of software differ from those of hardware

There are many more distinct paths to check in software, thus more areas where failures could be hidden

Repair of a hardware fault generally restores the system to its previous configuration, whereas repair of a software fault does not.

From these differences, it is apparent the job of designing quality software is a challenging one.

8.2 Software Reliability

Software reliability is defined as:

The probability of failure-free operation of a software

component or system in a specified environment for a specified period of time.

The goals of a software reliability program include:

Ease design and maintenance tasks

Avoid errors at all stages of development

Detect errors at the earliest possible time, when they are easiest and least expensive to fix.

Assure the software does not reduce the reliability of the device.

Figure 8.1 Software Development Costs

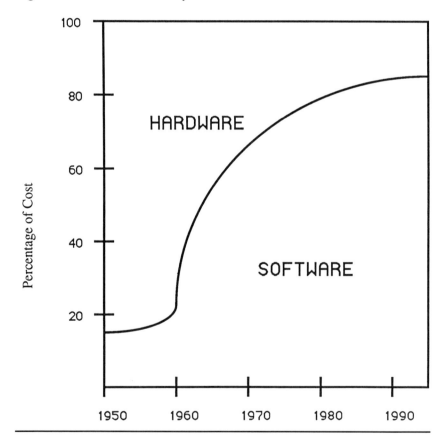

There are four reasons for assuring a reliable software design:

    Safety
    Cost
    The Market
    The FDA.

Safety is the most important reason for having reliable software. As with hardware, software failures must not have the potential to injure the user or patient. Liability cases are becoming more frequent and costly. A company cannot afford the risk if it wants to remain profitable.

Figure 8.2 Software Error Detection Cost

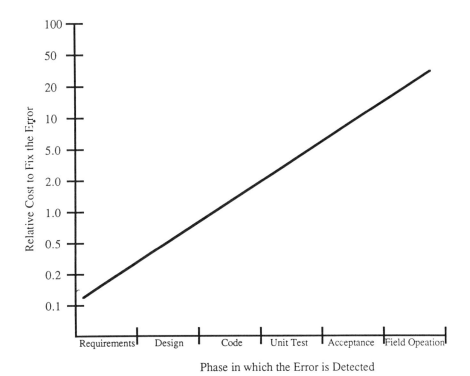

Cost has a dual impact on software development. The cost of software development as a percentage of the total development cost has steadily increased since 1955 (Figure 8.1). At that time, hardware development accounted for approximately 82% of the total development cost, while software accounted for approximately 18%. By 1985, due to technological advances in hardware and the increased functionality taken on by software, hardware development accounted for 18%, while software development development accounted for 82%. With the increased amount of time and money required for software development, it is important it be done right the first time. The more cost effective the design process, the less costly the overall product cost.

Cost also has an impact in error detection and correction. It has been estimated that it is 100 times more costly to catch and repair a "bug" in the field that it is to catch and repair it in the design phase (Figure 8.2). Cost are directly proportional to the point in the life cycle when the error is detected and repaired.

Software errors are costly in the marketplace. Disregarding any safety issues, software errors are not only an inconvenience to the customer, but serve to damage the reputation of the manufacturer. As the reputation suffers, so does the market share.

The fourth reason for reliable software is the FDA.

8.3 Software and the FDA

Within the past few years, the subject of software in and as medical devices has become an important topic for the FDA. This interest began in 1985 when software in a radiation treatment therapy device is alleged to have resulted in a lethal overdose. The FDA then analyzed recalls by fiscal year and determined how many were due to software problems. Figure 8.3 is a representative example of that analysis. In FY 1985, for example, 20% of all neurology recalls were attributable to software problems, while 8% of cardiovascular recalls had the same cause. This type of analysis along with the results of various inspections led the FDA to conclude that some type of regulation was required.

Since there are many types of software in use in the medical area, the problem of the best way to regulate it has become an issue for the FDA. Discussions have centered around what type of software is a medical device, the type of regulation required for such software and what could be inspected under current regulations.

A draft of a software policy was issued in September, 1987. The policy was a general statement of FDA thinking, including the definition of a medical device, establishment of a three class system for regulation

Figure 8.3 FDA Recall Data

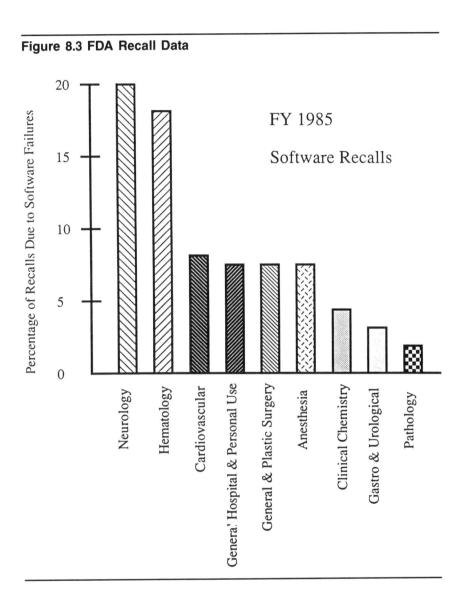

FY 1985

Software Recalls

and a list of exemptions from the regulations. The policy draft is very general and leaves much room for personal interpretation. The draft policy did not address GMP issues or the status of software as an inspectable commodity. As of this writing, the final policy has not been published.

The FDA has published guidelines for on developing quality software, the requirements for product approval submissions and the inspection of software controlled test fixtures as a part of a GMP inspection. The FDA has also conducted training courses for their inspectors on the subject of software and computer basics.

As of this writing, there are no published regulations giving the FDA the authority to inspect the design and development of software as a part of a GMP inspection, although it may not be long before such a regulation is enacted. Many individual inspectors have taken the guidelines to be the regulation and are inspecting to them. The problem is compounded by the fact that there is no Agency coordination of inspectors. Each inspector can inspect to his own philosophy of software quality assurance. Some companies have been shut down for a lack of what the inspector considered to be a proper software development process. Some companies have taken the FDA to court over this matter, without any general premise being established.

Organizations such as the Health Industry Manufacturers Association (HIMA) and the National Electronic Manufacturers Association (NEMA), have had active software taskforces in place for several years. These taskforces work with members, to meet with the FDA, discuss issues and present position papers on what industry feels the software policy should contain and what can be inspected during a normal GMP inspection. To facilitate this effort, HIMA and NEMA recently combined efforts in a joint taskforce that is instrumental in presenting the veiwpoint of the manufacturer to the FDA.

8.4 Software Quality Assurance

The term "Software Quality Assurance" (SQA) is defined as:

> A planned and systematic pattern of activities performed to assure the procedures, tools and techniques used during software development and modification are adequate to provide the desired level of confidence in the final product.

The purpose of the Software Quality Assurance program is to ensure that software is of such quality that it does not reduce the reliability of the device. Assurance that a product works reliably has been classically provided by a test of the product at the end of its development period. However, because of the nature of software, no test appears sufficiently comprehensive to adequately test all aspects of the program, especially when the length of some software programs exceeds five million lines of code. Therefore, Software Quality Assurance has taken the form of directing and documenting the development process itself, including checks and balances.

Activities included in the design phase, which serve to assure the quality of the software, include:

> Software specification
> A structured approach to the design
> Module Interaction
> Software reviews.

8.4.1 Software Specification

The software specification is the first step in the development of any software package. It is a detailed summary of what the software is to do and how it will do it. The specification should include:

> Functional requirements
> Review of the hardware
> Program flow diagrams
> Module definition
> Module interaction
> Memory map
> Data dictionary
> Interrupt handling
> Self diagnostics
> Hardware/software interface
> Error recovery
> Initialization.

The specification is written by the author(s) of the software program, based upon the requirements detailed in the Product Specification. The Software Specification should be as detailed as possible, in order to shorten the actual design and coding time. The Software Specification should also be a controlled document. Changes must go through the revision control process.

8.4.2 Structured Design

Once the specification is complete, a structured approach to the design can begin. The first activity includes the choice of a model for the software development. The choice may be a cascade model, where all activity is sequential. A device of lesser complexity, such as a digital thermometer or certain monitors, would be candidates for a cascade model.

As the complexity of the device increases, the design of certain modules may depend on the performance of previously designed modules. The cascade model is not applicable in this situation and the iterative model is a better candidate.

Another choice the designer must make is the type of structured approach, such as top down design or bottom up. The choice depends upon the intended application and the environment in which the software is to be used.

Top down design has become identified with good software practices. It works from major modules and breaks them into smaller, more manageable modules. It is a rational, systematic method which address problems characterized by a purely functional specification, known and frozen at the outset. One flaw in top down design is that it neglects the need for change and reuse.

Bottom up design starts from available components and builds on them. A good solution to a problem is produced, minimizing the effort by building on previous achievements and striving for the highest possible degree of generality to facilitate future developments. The goal is to produce components that may be combined in various ways, not favoring any of these ways during development.

The choice of a language is based on the intended use of the device and the ease with which the functionality can be programmed. The language chosen should be one which is easy to maintain.

The major choice in language is between high level languages and assembly languages. Where control of the functionality is a major concern, assembly language is the choice. Where functional control is not a priority a high level language may be chosen based on its ease of use.

8.4.3 Module Interaction

An important part of the software design, which is often overlooked or left to the last minute, is the definition of the requirements for different software modules to interface and work together. Many times, individual programmers are assigned the design and coding of individual modules. They may go about their business without any thought of how the other modules will interact with theirs. When all the modules are put together, the program doesn't work. A portion of the software specification should be devoted to defining the requirements for module interaction.

8.4.4 Software Reviews

Software reviews should be held at key stages of development, such as at completion of the specification, the design, the testing and the development process. This action presents fewer problems if coding has not begun, as corrections will be required only in the documentation. If coding has begun, corrections will be required in both the documentation and the program, which adds extra time and cost to the development. These reviews are scheduled in order to provide an unbiased look at the results of the activity and to offer suggestions for improvement.

A software review should be attended by three or four software personnel not involved with the program under scrutiny, but who are experienced in software design, the language being utilized and proper coding procedures. One member of Reliability Assurance should also be in attendance to assure the software, as designed, will not reduce the reliability of the device. All participants should have some familiarity with hardware design.

Any pertinent documentation, such as the specification, flow charts, data diagrams, etc. should be sent to each participant approximately one week in advance of the review. Participants are expected to review all material and develop a list of questions, pertinent to the review. A sample of such questions is given in Figure 8.4. Large software programs should be divided into segments, with each segment reviewed independently, within a close time frame.

All software reviews are governed by three strict rules: The material is reviewed, not the author; the focus is on the detection of errors, not corrective action; the review is held in an open, non-defensive atmosphere.

The actual review has a chairperson who directs the meeting. The chair is usually the Product Development Manager. A secretary is appointed and is responsible for documenting all discussions, all issues raised and all action items assigned. These activities are summarized in a set of review minutes, that become part of the product file.

The actual review is presented by the author(s) of the program and consists of an overview of the pertinent hardware, followed by a detailed walk-through of the software. Visual aids are suggested for ease of presentation. Constructive criticism is given by the reviewers and recorded by the secretary. All previously prepared questions are addressed. Action items are defined and documented.

Once issues have been raised and documented, the author(s) must address and validate each one. If the required corrections are extensive, another review may be necessary.

Figure 8.4 Sample Software Review Checklist

Software Review Checklist
Is the system initialized?
Can the initialization and/or system test be implemented without turning the unit off?
Is a RAM check included to assure the integrity of the RAM contents?
Is a variable check included to assure the software has not wandered off?
Is a checksum performed to assure the integrity of the software?
Is the display test format sufficient to have checked all segments?
Are self diagnostics implemented?
How does the program handle simultaneous inputs or interrupts?
What are the priorities on interrupts?
How does the software handle unspecified inputs?
Can the system be hung by activitating a wrong key or switch?
What happens if a software error occurs?
Are error messages clear and helpful?
Does the software contain diagnostic and debugging aids?
Are records kept of the inputs for later failure analysis or recovery needs?
Are there provisions for protection against singularities, such as division by zero?
Does the software contain a method for recovery, if a glitch or power loss occurs?

8.5 Software Safety

It has been argued that there is no such thing as software safety since software by itself cannot be unsafe. However, since software, by itself, is of little value to anyone other than a programmer, a broader system view is that software can have various unexpected and undesired effects when used in a complex system.

A system is:

The sum total of all its component parts, working together within a given environment, to achieve a given purpose or mission, within a given time, over a given life span.

The state of the system is made up of the state of the components of the system, one of which is a computer. Software safety then involves assuring that the software executes within the context of a system without resulting in unacceptable risk. What risk is acceptable or unacceptable must be defined for each system and often involves economic, political and moral decisions.

As with hardware safety, software safety is achieved by identifying potential hazards early in the development process and then establishing requirements and design features to eliminate or control these hazards.

System safety analysis procedures often start by defining what is hazardous and then working backward to find all combinations of faults that produce the event. The probability of occurrence of the event can then be calculated and the result evaluated as to acceptability. Potential hazards that need to be considered include:

Normal operating modes
Maintenance modes
System failure modes
Failures or unusual incidents in the environment
Errors in human performance.

There are several techniques used in software analysis, including:

Fault tree analysis
Real time logic
Time Petri nets.

Fault tree analysis is an analytical technique which can be used in the safety analysis of software systems. An undesired state is specified, and the system is then analyzed in the context of its environment and operation to find credible sequences of events that can lead to the undesired state. The fault tree is a graphic model of various parallel and sequential combinations of faults or system states that will result in the occurrence of the predefined undesired event. Faults can be events associated with component hardware failures, human errors, or other pertinent events. A fault tree depicts the logical interrelationships of basic events that lead to the hazardous event. Fault tree analysis is discussed in detail in Chapter 9.

Real time logic shows how to formalize the safety analysis of timing properties in real-time systems. The system designer first specifies a model of the system in terms of events and actions. The event-action model describes the data dependency and temporal ordering of the computational actions that must be taken in response to events in a real-time application. This model can be mechanically translated into real time logic formulas. In contrast to other forms of temporal logic specification, real time logic allows specification of the absolute timing of events, not only their relative ordering, and provides a uniform way of incorporating different scheduling disciplines in the inference mechanism.

Time Petri net models allow mathematical modeling of discrete-event systems in terms of conditions and events and the relationship between them. Analysis and simulation procedures have been developed to determine desirable and undesirable properties of the design, especially with respect to concurrent or parallel events. Analysis procedures have been developed to determine software safety requirements directly from the system, to analyze a design for safety, recoverability and fault tolerance and to guide in the use of failure detection and recovery procedures.

8.6 Software Metrics

Software must be subjected to measurement in order to achieve a true indication of quality and reliability. Quality attributes must be related to specific product requirements and must be quantified. This is accomplished through the use of metrics.

Metrics must be selected that:

> Are useful to the specific objectives of the program
>
> Have been derived from the program requirements
>
> Support the evaluation of the software consistent with the specified requirements.

To develop accurate estimates a historical baseline must be established consisting of data collected from previous software projects. The data collected must be:

Reasonably accurate

Collected from as many projects as possible

Consistent

Representative of applications that are similar to work that is to be estimated.

Once the data has been collected metric computation is possible. Depending on the breadth of the data, metrics can span a broad range of measures.

Two metrics that are typically used in software analysis are Mc Cabe's Complexity and Halstead Measures.

8.6.1 McCabe's Complexity

This metric relates a complexity to the measure of the structure of the software. It is derived from classical graph theory. The metric is described by the equation:

$$V(G) = e - n + 2p$$

where
$V(g)$ = complexity number
e = number of edges in the program
n = number of vertices
p = number of connected components.

As an example consider the software module in Figure 8.5.

Figure 8.5 Software Module

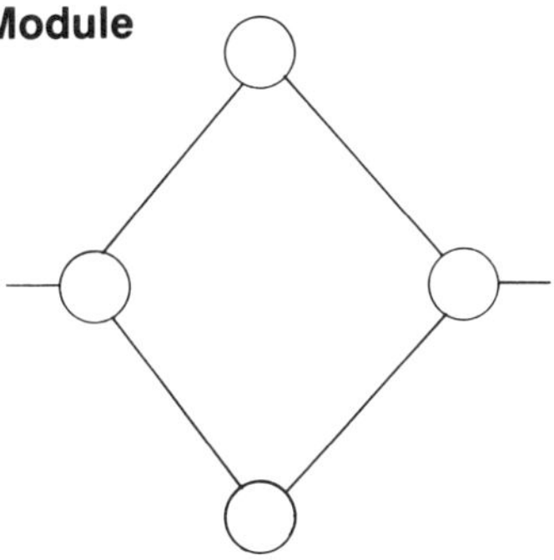

For the module:

$$e = 4; n = 4; p = 1$$

Thus,

$$V(G) = e - n + 2p$$
$$= 4 - 4 + 2(1)$$
$$= 2$$

The higher the complexity of the software module, the more difficult it will be to build, test and maintain.

8.6.2 Halstead Measures

These metrics provide a measure of the quality of the software development process by accounting for two factors: the number of distinct operators (instruction types) and the number of distinct operands (variables and constraints). Halstead defines a number of characteristics that can be quantified about the software and then relates these in different ways to describe the various aspects of the software. Three such measures are:

> Vocabulary of the software
> Length of the program
> Volume of the software.

8.6.2.1 Vocabulary of the Software

This measure is defined as:

$$n = n1 + n2$$

where

$n1$ = the number of distinct operators
$n2$ = the number of distinct operands.

8.6.2.2 Length of the Program

This measure is defined as:

$$N = N1 + N2$$

where

$N1$ = the total number of occurrences of operators
$N2$ = the total number of occurrences of operands.

8.6.2.3 Volume of Software

This measure is defined as:

$$V = N \log_2 n$$

where

N = length of the program
n = vocabulary of the software.

8.6.3 Other Metrics

Other metric techniques have been developed that measure the total process of the software development through a complete set of attribute descriptors including:

Complexity
Correctness
Efficiency
Flexibility
Integrity
Interoperability
Maintainability
Portability
Testability
Usability.

8.6.4 Computer Aided Metrics

There are programs currently available which will analyze a software program by module and produce metric measurements. These measurements include call graphs, Kiviat diagrams of metric measurements and module maps which indicate the number of entrances, exits and statement types within a module. These graphic measurements are particularly useful in reviewing revision level changes to the software and their effect on each module.

8.7 Software Failures

To understand how to avoid software errors, it is necessary to understand what causes software failures. Software doesn't degrade like hardware and it is not constrained physically. Therefore, the causes of software failures are significantly different from those of hardware components.

There are four causes of software failures:

Specification errors
Design errors
Typographical errors
Omissions of symbols.

Specification errors are caused by a misunderstanding of the customer's real needs. Many programs have been developed with the customer's needs in mind, only to find out later the device did not function as the customer expected it to. There must be a genuine effort to fully understand what the customers need and what they expect the device to do.

Design errors are probably the most frequent cause of software errors. The designer, after reviewing the specification, may be more interested in starting to code, rather than spending time thinking through the design. This practice may lead to decision points within the program not addressing all conditions or to the establishment of race conditions.

Typographical errors are the third cause of failures. When keying the code, it is easy to hit a wrong key or copy the code improperly. An example of such an error having a costly effect is the delay, just prior to launch, of a space shuttle flight. The software shut the system down with less than a minute until launch. Analysis traced the cause to a typographical error of a DO statement, where the DO was followed by a variable name. When keyed, the space between the DO and the variable name was omitted, causing the program to consider the whole line as a variable name. When the variable name was not recognized, the software shut the system down.

Another cause of software errors, similar to typographical errors, is the omission of symbols. When symbols are omitted, the code becomes unrecognizable and the program will fail.

As the causes of software errors are understood, methods can be employed to eliminate such causes, thereby eliminating the failures. This puts the emphasis of the Software Quality Assurance program on avoidance of errors, rather than detection of errors, making for a more reliable program, more quickly.

8.8 Coding

Coding of the program occurs after the software specification review has been completed and the design finalized. If the specification is complete and the design has been properly structured, coding time will be minimized as modules and module interfaces fall into place within the structure of the program.

Coding should begin at the lowest or module level. When all modules have been coded, the next level is the module interfaces and then the main program. By moving from the lowest to the highest level, activity can be completed most effectively.

As coding proceeds, authors, working with Quality Assurance, should be planning a test protocol that validates the code they are producing, in as many paths as practically possible. The test should be structured such that all areas of the program are exercised and evaluated and all combinations of multiple inputs are included.

8.9 Summary

Software in and as a medical device is subjected to a software quality assurance program to assure safety is designed in, to reduce costs, to provide a reliable medical device in the market place and to satisfy FDA requirements. The program consists of developing a software specification, establishing a structured approach to the design, conducting software reviews at appropriate times and defining software failures for the particular device and its intended application. A concerted effort in the design will reduce coding time.

8.10 References

1. ANSI/IEEE Standard 729, *IEEE Standard Glossary of Software Engineering Terminology*. New York: The Institute of Electrical and Electronic Engineers, 1983.

2. ANSI/IEEE Standard 730, *IEEE Standard for Software Quality Assurance Plans*. New York: The Institute of Electrical and Electronic Engineers, 1984.

3. ANSI/IEEE Standard 828, *IEEE Standard for Software Configuration Management Plans*. New York: The Institute of Electrical and Electronic Engineers, 1983.

4. ANSI/IEEE Standard 830, *IEEE Guide to Software Requirements*

Specifications. New York: The Institute of Electrical and Electronic Engineers, 1984.

5. ANSI/IEEE Standard 983, *IEEE Guide for Software Quality Assurance Planning*. New York: The Institute of Electrical and Electronic Engineers, 1986.

6. ANSI/IEEE Standard 1016, *IEEE Recommended Practice for Software Design Descriptions*. New York: The Institute of Electrical and Electronic Engineers, 1987.

7. Arthur, L.J., *Measuring Programmer Productivity and Software Quality*. New York: John Wiley and Sons, 1984.

8. Boehm, B. W., "Software Engineering," *IEEE Transactions on Computers*. Volume C-25, Number 12, December, 1976.

9. Boehm, B. W., *Software Engineering Economics*. Englewood Cliffs, New Jersey: Prentice-Hall Incorporated, 1981.

10. Boehm, B. W., "A Spiral Model of Software Development and Enhancement," *Computer*. May, 1988.

11. Dean, E. S., "Software System Safety," *Proceedings of the 5th International System Safety Conference*. Volume 1, Part 1, Newport Beach, California: System Safety Society, 1981.

12. DHSS, *Functional Safety of Programmable Electronic Systems: Generic Aspects*. 1987

13. Dunn, R., *Software Defect Removal*. New York: McGraw-Hill Book Company, 1984.

14. IEEE Standard 796, *IEEE Standard Microcomputer System Bus*. New York: The Institute of Electrical and Electronic Engineers, 1983.

15. IEEE Standard 1058.1, *IEEE Standard for Software Project Management Plans*. New York: The Institute of Electrical and Electronic Engineers, 1987.

16. IEEE Standard 1063, *IEEE Standard for Software User Documentation*. New York: The Institute of Electrical and Electronic Engineers, 1987.

17. FDA, *Guide to the Inspection of Computerized Systems in Drug Processing*. 1983.

18. FDA, *Process Control Systems* (FDA Training Program). 1985.

19. FDA, *FDA Policy for the Regulation of Computer Products* (Draft). 1987.

20. FDA, *Software Development Activities.* 1987

21. FDA, *Medical Device GMP Guidance for FDA Investigators.* 1987

22. FDA, *Reviewer Guidance for Computer-Controlled Medical Devices* (Draft). 1988.

23. Fairly, R. E., *Software Engineering Concepts.* New York: McGraw-Hill Book Company, 1985.

24. Fries, R. C. and P. W. Heide, "Establishing a Software Quality Assurance Program for Microprocessor-based Medical Equipment," *Medical Instrumentation.* Volume 20, Number 3, May-June, 1986.

25. Fries, R. C. and P. W. Heide, "A Software Quality Assurance Procedure for Microprocessor-Based Medical Equipment," *Biomedical Technology Today.* September-October, 1986.

26. Fries, R. C., J. A. Roberts and J. M. Leen, "Practical Software Reliability," *Proceedings of the AAMI 21st Annual Meeting.* 1986.

27. Garwood, R. M., "FDA's Viewpoint on Inspection of Computer Systems," *HIMA Conference on the Regulation of Medical Software Proceedings.* 1987.

28. Holstein, H., "FDA Access to Device Software Research Documentation," *Proceedings from the HIMA Conference, FDA Regulation of Medical Software.* 1988.

29. Jahanian, F. and A. K. Mok, "Safety Analysis of Timing Properties in Real-Time Systems," *IEEE Transactions on Software Engineering.* Volume SE-12, Number 9, September, 1986.

30. Jorgens III, J. and C. W. Burch, "FDA Regulation of Computerized Medical Devices," *Byte.* Volume 7, 1982.

31. Jorgens III, J., "Computer Hardware and Software as Medical Devices," *Medical Device and Diagnostic Industry.* May, 1983.

32. Jorgens III, J. and R. Schneider, "Regulation of Medical Software by the FDA," *Software in Health Care.* April-May, 1985.

33. Kahan, J. S., "Regulation of Computer Hardware and Software as Medical Devices," *Canadian Computer Law Reporter*. Volume 4, Number 3, January, 1987.

34. Leveson, N. G., "Software Safety: Why, What and How," *Computing Surveys*. Volume 18, Number 2, June, 1986.

35. Lloyd, D. K. and M. Lipow, *Reliability Management, Methods and Mathematics*. 2nd Edition, Milwaukee, Wisconsin: The Anerican Society for Quality Control, 1984.

36. McCabe, T., "A Complexity Measure," *IEEE Transactions of Software Engineering*. SE-2, Number 4, December, 1976.

37. Musa, J. D., "The Measurement and Management of Software, Reliability," *Proceedings of the IEEE*. Volume 68, 1980.

38. Musa, J. D., *Software Reliability*. New York: Mc Graw-Hill Book Company, 1987.

39. Myers, G. J., *The Art of Software Testing*. New York: John Wiley and Sons, 1979.

40. Peterson, J. L., *Petri Net Theory and the Modeling of Systems*. Englewood Cliffs, New Jersey: Prentice-Hall, 1981.

41. Pressman, R., *Software Engineering*. New York: Mc Graw-Hill Book Company, 1987.

42. TUV Study Group on Conputer Safety, *Microcomputers in Safety Technique—An Aid to Orientation for Developers and Manufacturers*. 1987.

43. Unknown, "Quality: the Competitive Edge," *Focus*. February, 1988.

44. Vesely, W. E. et al., *Fault Tree Handbook*. U. S. Nuclear Regulatory Commission, 1981.

9

The Validation Phase Hardware

The heart of the product development process is the validation phase. During this phase testing indicates how well the product has been designed. The initial parts count reliability predication had indicated whether the design would meet the reliability goal and what parts of the circuit had the potential for high failure rate. It did not give an indication of how the parts would work together once the device became operational. To obtain this information, testing must be performed with the device operating in its intended application, as well as in the worst case environment.

9.1 The Test

Validation testing can be defined as subjecting a device to conditions that show its character or lack of character. Throughout the development cycle testing is done to provide pertinent information to the development team. Because the types of information required change during the various development stages, different testing techniques must be employed.

The hardware is a factor in determining the type of test, the purpose of the test, and the length of time required to accomplish the test. Testing may be performed for various reasons:

Vendor evaluation
Vendor comparison
Component limitability
Failure mode analysis
Enviromental stress
Product use/misuse
Reliability demonstration.

Testing is performed in either a standard or an accelerated mode. In the standard mode, tests are run at ambient temperature and typical usage parameters. The test time is the actual time of operation. In the accelerated mode, test time is reduced by varying parameters, such as temperature, voltage or frequency of cycling, above their normal levels, or performing a test, such as sudden death testing. More will be said about these later in the chapter.

9.2 Test Protocol

It has been said that testing without a plan is not testing at all, but an experiment. It is essential that each test performed be detailed in a test plan. The test plan should include:

> The device
> The type of test
> The purpose of the test
> Definition of each failure
> Special requirements, as applicable
> The number of units on test
> Length of the test
> A detailed procedure specific to the component or device
> The parameters to be recorded.

9.2.1 Type of Test

Various types of test are conducted to determine the equipment's weaknesses, behavior characteristics and modes of failure. Testing can be categorized into four types:

> Long term reliabity testing
> Event Testing
> Overstress Testing
> Environmental Testing.

9.2.1.1 Long Term Reliability Testing

Long term reliability testing is conducted primarily to determine parameters, such as failure rate and Mean Time Between Failure. Long term reliability testing can also be conducted to determine what part or component fails, when it fails, the mode of failure at that particular time, the mechanism of failure and how much more or less life the equipment has that is required for operational use. This allows priorities of criticality for reliability improvement to be established.

9.2.1.2 Event Testing

Event testing consists of repeated testing of equipment through its cycle of operation until failure. This type of testing is analogous to time-to-failure testing. One important parameter developed from this type of test is the number of cycles to failure.

9.2.1.3 Overstress Testing

Overstress testing has an important place in reliability assessment, but care must be taken in its application. Too much overstress may make the test results inconclusive. Care should also be taken to overstress in steps, rather than attempting to get to the maximum value immediately. If the device fails, the step method allows the determination of where in the progression the failure occurred.

9.2.1.4 Environmental Testing

Environmental testing represents a survey of the reaction of a device to the enviromental and shipping environments it will experience in its daily usage. By investigating a broad spectrum of the environmental space, greater confidence is developed in the equipment than if it was merely subjected to ambient conditions. As with overstress testing, avoid unusually extreme or unrealistic environmental levels because of the difficulty in the interpretation of the results.

9.2.1.5 Other Types of Testing

There are two additional types of tests, based on the mode in which the test is conducted:

> Time related
> Failure related.

9.2.1.5.1 Time Related

Time related testing is conducted until a certain number of hours of operation or a certain number of cycles has been completed, e.g., a switch test conducted for 100,000 ON/OFF cycles or a monitor operated for 100,000 hours.

9.2.1.5.2 Failure Related

A test may be conducted until all test units or a certain percentage of units have failed, e.g., ventilators operated until the first unit fails or power supplies power cycled until all have failed.

These two types of tests will be important in choosing the correct formula to calculate MTBF from the test data.

9.2.2 Purpose of the Test

There are several purposes for testing:

> Feasibility of a design
> Comparing two or more vendors
> Comparing two or more configurations
> Testing the response to environmental stresses
> Developing reliability parameters
> Failure analysis.

All testing, except the reliability demonstration which is performed at the end of the product development cycle, is performed at a confidence level of 90%. This means one is 90% confident that the reliability parameters established in the test will be characteristic of units in the field. A 90% confidence level also yields a risk factor of (1 − the confidence level) or 10%. The reliability demonstration should be conducted at a confidence level of 95%, giving a risk factor of 5%. These levels will be important in determining the number of test units and the length of test time.

9.2.3 Failure Definition

For each test and for each device, a failure must be defined. This definition depends on the intended application and the anticipated environment. What is considered a failure for one component or device may not be a failure for another. The test protocol should be as detailed as possible in defining the failure.

9.2.4 Determining Sample Size and Test Length

Once you determine the type of test to be performed, you need to decide on the test sample size and the length of time necessary to accomplish your testing goal. Sample size and test time are dependent upon the MTBF goal, originally defined in the Product Specification, and on the confidence level at which the test will be conducted.

The formula for determining the sample size and test time is derived from the following equation:

MTBF goal = (sample size)(test time) $(2)/X^2_{\alpha;\ 2r\ +\ 2}$

where test time refers to the number of hours or the number of cycles the test will be conducted.

The equation thus becomes:

(sample size)(test time) = MTBF goal $(X^2_{\alpha;\ 2r\ +\ 2})/2$

where

α = the risk level = 1 − confidence level

r = number of failures

To complete the equation, we must first understand the Chi Square chart, included in Appendix 1. To use this chart, first find the risk level that the chart is based upon. As mentioned earlier, the risk factor is derived from the confidence level:

Confidence level = 1 − α

where

α = risk level

Thus, a confidence level of 90% yields a risk factor of 10%, while a confidence level of 95% yields a risk factor of 5%.

When calculating sample size and test time, it is assumed there will be no failures. The equation thus becomes:

(sample size)(test time) = (MTBF goal)$(X^2_{\alpha;\ 2})/2$

Looking at the Chi Square chart in Appendix 1, go across the top row of the chart and find 0.10, or $\propto$. Go down that column to the line for ν = 2, or (2r + 2). There you will find the number 4.605, or 4.61. Put this into the equation:

(sample size)(test time) = MTBF goal (4.61)/2

When you insert the MTBF goal, the product of sample size and test time is calculated. To determine each individual value, use the following law of statistics:

1 unit tested for 1000 hours is statistically equal to 10 units tested for 100 hours each is statistically equal to 50 units tested for 20 hours each.

Example 9.1

We want to test some monitors to prove a MTBF goal of 8760 hours of operation. How many units do we test and for how long, assuming no failures?

(sample size)(test time) = MTBF goal (4.61)/2

(sample size)(test time) = 8760 (4.61)/2

$$= 20192$$

From this data, we can calculate the following possibilities:

Sample Size	Test Time (hours)
1	20192
5	4038
10	2019
15	1346
20	1010
25	808

Example 9.2

We want to test monitors to prove the MTBF goal of 8760 hours of operation. How many units do we test and for how long, assuming one failure?

(sample size)(test time) = MTBF goal $(X^2_{\alpha; 2r + 2})/2$

$$= 8760 \ (7.779)/2$$

$$= 34072$$

We can then calculate:

Sample Size	Test Time (hours)
1	34072
5	6814
10	3407
15	2771
20	1704
25	1363

An interesting observation is that one failure increased the test time by 69%. A second failure would yield the equation:

(sample size)(test time) = 8760 (10.645)/2

$$= 46625$$

This is an increase in time of 37% over the one failure example and 131% over zero failures. This proves that unreliability is costly in time and effort.

9.2.5 Sample Test Protocol

The protocol should be reviewed by the Product Development Manager and the Reliability Assurance Manager and approved by signature when no further changes to the protocol are necessary. This assures both groups agree on the test and what it is to accomplish. Figure 9.1 shows a sample test protocol sheet. Figure 9.2 shows a completed protocol.

Figure 9.1 Sample Test Protocol

Reliability Assurance Test Protocol

Product	Unit Under Test	
Test Start Date	Lab Book Reference	Test Type

Test Procedure:

Day/Time to be Checked:

Checkout Procedure:

Reliability Technician	Date

Approvals

Product Development Manager	Date	Reliability Assurance Manager	Date

Figure 9.2 Completed Test Protocol

Reliability Assurance Test Protocol

Product Model 3322 Monitor		Unit Under Test ON/OFF Switch
Test Start Date 6/13/87	Lab Book Reference 1021	Test Type Cycle Test

Test Procedure: A cycle consists of once in the ON state and once in the OFF state. Switches
are cycled at a rate of 5 cycles per minute. Each ON is represented by a green LED, each OFF
is represented by a red LED. The number of cycles completed is recorded on a counter.
The test will end when one million cycles have been completed or when all units have failed.

Day/Time to be Checked:
                 Daily at 8:00, 12:00 and 5:00
Checkout Procedure:
Check each LED for 5 cycles of operation. Assure all LEDs are lit appropriately. Record any
failures in the notebook with the number of cycles completed until failure.

Reliability Technician	Date

Approvals

Product Development Manager	Date	Reliability Assurance Manager	Date

One advantage of using such a form is that a copy can be placed in the
area where the test is being conducted. Anyone in the test area could
look at the protocol and be aware of what is being done. The protocol
also helps reliabilty technicians. When one may be out of the lab and
another must monitor the test. the protocol indicates what is being done
and what activity is necessary at any particular time.

9.3 Standard Tests

Standard tests are conducted at room temperature, with no acceleration of any parameters. Standard tests are varied, dependent upon their purpose, and include:

Cycle testing
Typical use testing
10 × 10 testing
Fault tree analysis
Failure modes and effects analysis
Environmental tests.

9.3.1 Cycle Testing

Cycle testing is usually conducted on individual components, such as switches, phone jacks or cable. Testing consists of placing the component in alternating states, such as ON and OFF for a switch or IN and OUT for a phone plug, while monitoring the operation in each state. One cycle consists of one pass through each state.

Cycle testing could consist of passing through the state of operation and non-operation of a component or device. Thus a power supply could be power-cycled, with a cycle consisting of going from zero power to maximum power and back to zero. For devices, a cycle could consist of eight hours ON and 16 hours OFF.

9.3.2 Typical Use Testing

Typical use testing consists of operation of a device in its typical environment. This testing is usually incorporated when conducting a reliability demonstration or for calculating a long term MTBF value.

The test unit is tested electrically and mechanically prior to testing. Certain parameters are checked at periodic times, such as 2, 4, 8, 24, 48, 72, 96 and 128 hours after beginning the test and weekly thereafter. These recordings aid in determining drift or degradation in certain parameters.

9.3.3 10 x 10 Testing

Ten samples of a component or device are subjected to a test where recordings of a particular parameter are taken at 10 different time periods. A chart is created with the ten units listed in the left column and the ten recordings listed across the top (Figure 9.3). Mean and standard deviation values are calculated for each of the ten recordings and ten units.

Figure 9.3 10 x 10 Test

Unit	1	2	3	4	5	6	7	8	9	10	Mean	S.D.
1	350	380	400	360	340	370	330	340	360	340	357	20
2	200	130	190	200	130	150	250	230	240	160	188	41
3	270	250	270	240	300	230	330	330	300	350	287	39
4	270	140	160	170	160	140	430	130	130	130	186	90
5	230	180	170	150	260	240	210	230	240	210	212	33
6	280	180	70	390	300	210	400	440	370	230	287	110
7	180	210	270	190	210	170	170	270	190	200	206	34
8	190	220	180	190	170	190	200	120	170	130	176	29
9	200	180	160	180	200	120	90	170	140	170	161	33
10	230	190	260	180	290	170	280	220	260	170	225	43
Mean	240	206	213	225	236	199	269	248	240	209		
S.D.	50	66	85	78	67	67	100	95	80	74		

By reading the horizontal rows of data, the repeatability of the results can be determined. By analyzing the vertical columns, the variability among the units can be measured.

9.3.4 Fault Tree Analysis

Fault tree analysis is a "paper analysis" type of testing. Analysis starts by considering the various system modes of failures and working downward to identify the component cause of the failure and the probability of that failure.

A fault tree is a logic diagram of a system that pictorially shows all probable failure modes and the sequence in which they occur, leading to a specified system failure. Since a logic flow process is used, standard logic and event symbols are used (Figure 9.4).

Figure 9.4 Logic Symbols

Event Symbols

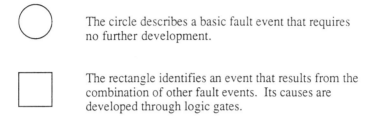

The circle describes a basic fault event that requires no further development.

The rectangle identifies an event that results from the combination of other fault events. Its causes are developed through logic gates.

The diamond depicts a secondary basic event, a composite of distinct failure events, not to be resolved in the fault tree.

Logic Gates

The AND gate describes the logical operation whereby the coexistence of all input events is required to produce the output event.

$$P4 = P1 \cdot P2 \cdot P3$$

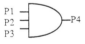

The OR gate describes the logical operation whereby the output event will exist if any or all of the input events exist.

$$P4 = P1 + P2 + P3 - (P1P2 + P1P3 + P2P3) + (P1 \cdot P2 \cdot P3)$$

9.3.4.1 The Fault Tree Process

Fault tree analysis is a stepwise sequential process beginning with the collection of appropriate documentation for creating the fault tree. This documentation may include parts lists, operating environment requirements, user manual, etc.

Once the documentation is reviewed, a failure is chosen that becomes the top event on the tree. This is the starting point for analysis and should be well defined and measurable. Where more than one top event can be identified, a separate fault tree should be conducted for each event.

Once this top event is identified, the fault tree can be developed. Branches from the top event are drawn to the events on the next level that could cause it. The secondary events are analyzed to determine if they are OR gates, AND gates or can be represented by an event symbol. The analysis continues downward until the lowest level is composed of basic fault events.

Once the tree is drawn, probability values are assigned to each gate or event. The quantification of the basic fault events can be derived from established sources of conponent failure rates, e.g., MIL-HDBK-217, field use failure data or vendor test data. Upper levels are calculated using the equations for the particular gates.

Finally, the analysis is reviewed to determine where corrective action is necessary. Once corrective action is decided upon, action items are assigned and completion dates set. Following the review, a summary test report is issued.

Figure 9.5 Alarm Circuit

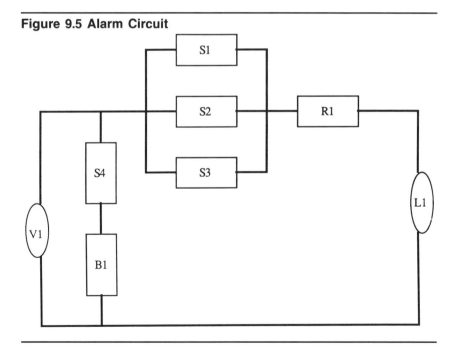

Example 9.3

An alarm circuit (Figure 9.5) is to be analyzed. Components and their probability of failure are shown in Figure 9.6.

Figure 9.6 Components and Failure Probabilities

Designation	Component	Failure Probability
S1	Switch	0.00438
S2	Switch	0.00438
S3	Switch	0.00438
R1	Resistor	0.00263
L1	Lamp	0.00876
V1	Volt Source	0.01752
S4	Switch	0.00438
B1	Battery	0.03679

The top event is chosen to be the lamp (C5) failing to light. The lamp would fail to light if:

the switches failed to close, or

the source failed, or

the lamp or resistor failed.

The next level of failures is chosen. The source fails if:

the voltage source is dead, or

the emergency battery is ineffective.

Figure 9.7 Fault Tree of the Alarm Circuit

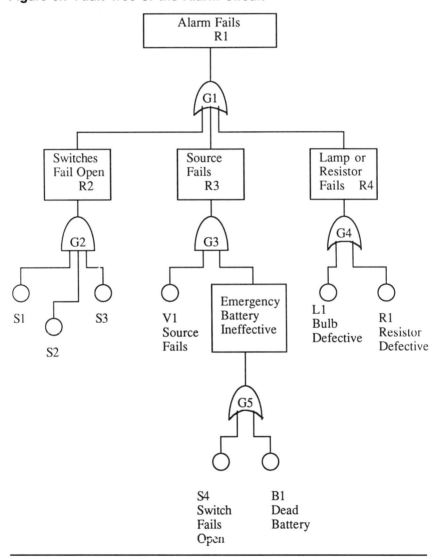

The lamp and resistor fails if:

the bulb is defective, or

the resistor is defective.

At the lowest level, the emergency battery is ineffective if:

the switch fails to close, or
the battery is dead.

Figure 9.8 Probability Tree

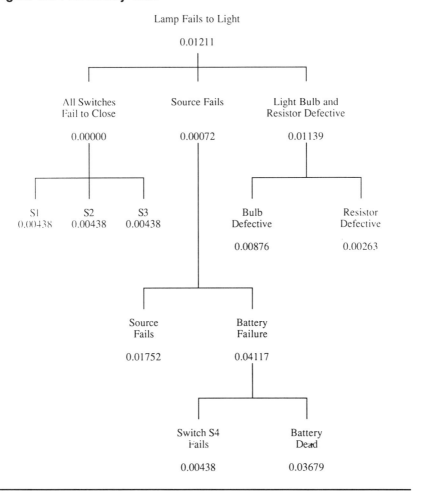

Once the fault tree is developed, the probabilities for each level can be entered in a probability tree and the probability of failure for the top event calculated, using the equations for the gates. Figure 9.8 shows the probability tree for the alarm circuit.

9.3.5 Failure Modes and Effects Analysis

Failure Modes and Effects Analysis (FMEA) is a test conducted to determine the effect of a single point failure on the output of the device. For devices where the circuitry is not extensive, the test is conducted on all components of the device. Where circuitry is extensive, the circuitry is reviewed by Reliability Assurance and Design Engineering to determine which portions are the most prone to failure or have a high failure rate. All components within these portions are subjected to testing.

The test is conducted on a breadboard of the circuitry or on an actual device, where all integrated circuits on the PC boards are socketed. The device is tested electrically and mechanically to assure it is operating according to specification.

During the test, the output of the device is continuously monitored. While monitoring the output, the following actions are taken:

Short each component, except integrated circuits.

Open each component.

Place 100K shunts to each component.

Open all pins on each integrated circuit.

Vary appropriate components to their plus and minus tolerances.

Input harmonics of the clocks and oscillators.

Vary input power plus and minus 10%, in 0.5 volt increments.

Short and shunt close neighboring tracks.

Short any tracks along the edge of the PC board.

Record any changes to the output for each failure mode applied to each component. Be especially aware of changes that could be safety hazards, such as increased voltages or defeat of the alarm system. For harmonic input and voltage variation, special attention should be given to the effect on the microprocessors and other integrated circuits.

A record is kept of each application of a failure mode. The record should contain the component acted upon, the failure mode (short, open, 100K shunt) and the effect observed. Figure 9.9 shows an example of the format of such a record. Figure 9.10 is a sample record.

Figure 9.9 FMEA Format

Failure Mode and Effects Analysis

Product:	Circuit Tested:
Date:	Tester:

Component	Failure Mode	Effect

Figure 9.10 Sample FMEA Record

Failure Mode and Effects Analysis

Product:	Circuit Tested:
Model 4255 Cardiac Monitor	Display Board
Date:	Tester:
11/3/88	James Roberts, CQT

Component	Failure Mode	Effect
U 112		
Pin 1	Open	Display comes on in a random pattern and then goes blank
Pin 2	Open	Display flickers. Does not return to normal after 5 minutes of operation.
Pin 3	Open	Operates normally
Pin 4	Open	Display is blank and remains so.
CR 12	Short	Display is not operative
	100K Shunt	Operates normally

All issues relating to safety must be addressed as soon as they are found. If a design change results, test the device again to assure the concern has been satisfactorily addressed. Concerns that do not involve safety should be evaluated on a risk and a cost basis.

A summary should be written highlighting the test results that have been addressed by the product team. If work sheets are few in number, include them in the test report. Otherwise, reference the location of the worksheets in the report.

The results of the Failure Modes and Effects Analysis are a valuable tool to share with the Service department. The list of effects by component failure mode will assist the Service Representatives in troubleshooting field failures and determining on the required action.

9.4 Accelerated Testing

Accelerated testing is a shortening of the length of the test time by varying the parameters of the test. Testing can be accelerated in several ways:

> Increase the sample size
> Increase the test severity
> Use sudden death testing.

9.4.1 Increasing Sample Size

Reliability tests are accelerated by increasing the sample size, provided the life distribution does not show a wearout characteristic during the anticipated life. Test time is inversely proportional to the sample size, so that increasing the sample size reduces the test time.

Large sample size reliability tests conducted to provide a high total operating time should be supported by some long duration tests if there is a reason to suspect that failure modes exist which have high times to failure.

9.4.2 Increasing Test Severity

Increasing test severity is a logical approach to reducing test time when large sample sizes cannot be used.

The severity of tests may be increased by increasing the stresses acting on the test unit. These stresses can be grouped into two categories:

> Operational, such temperature and humidity

> Application, such as voltage, current, self- generated heat or self-generated mechanical stresses

Increasing the temperature severity is the usual method of accelerating testing.

It is important, in accelerated testing, to assure that unrealistic failure modes are not introduced by the higher stresses. It is also possible that interactions may occur between separate stresses, so that the combined weakening effect is greater that would be expected from a single additive process.

When conducting accelerated testing, an essential calculation is acceleration factor, that is the parameter that indicates how much acceleration was conducted. To calculate the acceleration factor, the following equation is used:

Acceleration Factor = $\exp(-(EA/K)(1/TU - 1/TA))$
where
EA = Energy of Activation (0.5 eV)
K   = Boltzman's Constant (0.0000863 eV/degree Kelvin)
TU = Use temperature in degrees Kelvin
TA = Accelerate temperature in degrees Kelvin

Example 9.4

Ten units are tested to failure at 150 degrees Centigrade. The units are expected to be used at 85 degrees Centigrade. What is the minimum life (time of the first failure) at 85 degrees Centigrade? What is the MTBF at 85 degrees Centigrade?

The failure rates in hours are listed as:

2750	3100	3400	3800	4100
4400	4700	5100	5700	6400

Calculation of Acceleration Factor:
EA = 0.5
K   = 0.0000863
TU = 85 + 273 = 358 degrees Kelvin
TA = 150 = 273 = 423 degrees Kelvin

Acceleration factor = $\exp((-0.5/0.0000863)(1/358 - 1/423))$

$$= 12$$

Calculation of Minimum Life at 85 degrees Centigrade:

Minimum life = (acceleration factor) × (failure at 85 degrees)

$$= (12) \times (2750)$$

$$= 33,000 \text{ hours}$$

Calculation of MTBF at 150 degrees Centigrade:

MTBF = sum of the times of operation/number of errors

= 2750+3100+3400+3800+4100+4400+4700+5100
+5700+6400/10

= 43450/10

= 4345 hours

Calculation of MTBF at 85 degrees Centigrade:

MTBF = acceleration factor (MTBF at 150 degrees)

= 12 (4345)

= 52,140 hours

Example 9.5

Integrated circuits are to be burned-in to eliminate infant mortality failures. The burn-in is to be equivalent to 1000 hours of operation at ambient temperature (24 degrees Centigrade). How long do we run the units at 50 degrees Centigrade? How long do we run the units at 100 degrees Centigrade?

Calculation at 50 degrees Centigrade:

$$\text{Acceleration factor} = \exp(-0.5/0.0000863)(1/297 - 1/323)$$

$$= 4.8$$

$$\text{Length of run time} = \text{run time at 24 degrees/acceleration factor}$$

$$= 1000/4.8$$

$$= 208 \text{ hours}$$

Calculation at 100 degrees Centigrade:

$$\text{Acceleration factor} = \exp((-0.5/0.0000863)(1/297 - 1/373))$$

$$= 53$$

$$\text{Length of time} = 1000/53$$

$$= 19 \text{ hours}$$

9.4.3 Sudden Death Testing

Sudden Death testing is a form of accelerated testing where the total test sample is arbitrarily divided into several, equally-numbered groups.

All units in each group are started simultaneously. When the first unit in a group fails, the whole group is considered to have failed. Testing is stopped on the remaining unfailed units in the group as soon as the first one fails. The entire test is terminated when the first unit in the last group fails.

Sudden Death testing is conducted using Weibull Analysis.

9.4.3.1 Weibull Analysis

The Weibull distribution was first introduced in 1949 by W. Weibull of Sweden as a convenient method of analyzing mechanical fatigue data. Since its introduction, it has been used extensively in areas such as bearing fatigue data and prediction about the failure of automotive parts.

The Weibull distribution has properties which permit it to be fitted to many kinds of data. This results in wide confidence intervals as increased generality results in decreased precision. The distribution uses three parameters:

> The scale parameter - alpha
> The shape parameter - beta
> The location parameter - gamma

The scale parameter controls the amount of skewness or spreading from left to right. The shape parameter controls the shape of the distribution function. The location parameter establishes the position of the left end of the distribution and is usually considered to be zero.

The shape parameter (beta) is indicative of the portion of the life cycle the data represents. Where beta is less than one, the data is indicative of the infant mortality period of the life cycle. Where beta is equal to one, the data is indicative of the useful life period. Where beta is greater than one, the data is indicative of the wearout period of the life cycle.

Weibull paper is a logarithmic probability plotting paper constructed with the y-axis representing the cumulative probability of failure and the x-axis representing a time value, in hours or cycles.

Data points are established from failure data, with the failure times arranged in increasing order or value of occurrence. Corresponding median ranks are assigned from a percent rank table, based on the sample size. An example will illustrate the point:

Example 9.6

Six power supplies were placed on life test. The six units failed at 150,

85, 175, 280, 350 and 225 hours respectively. To plot the data, first arrange the failure times in increasing value, as listed below. Then determine the median ranks by using the table in Appendix 2, with N = sample size = 6. Going to the column headed by 50.0, read the six median ranks as below:

Failure Order Number	Life in Hours	Median Ranks (%)
1	45	10.910
2	100	26.445
3	170	42.141
4	240	57.859
5	340	73.555
6	530	89.090

Figure 9.11 shows the resultant plot. The resultant line can be used to determine the MTBF and the percent that will fail at any given time. For $\beta = 1$, the MTBF is found by drawing a line from the 63.2% point on the y-axis to the resultant line. Then, dropping a line from this point to the x-axis gives the MTBF value. From the plot, the MTBF is 262 hours.

To find the percentage of units that will have failed at 1000 hours, draw a vertical line from the x-axis to the resultant line. Then draw a horizontal line from that point to the y-axis. This is the failure percentage. In this case, 99.2% of all units produced will fail by 1000 hours.

9.4.3.2 Confidence Limits

The confidence limits for this example can be determined in a similar fashion. For example, if the 90% confidence level for the above test were desired, the 5% and 95% ranks would be obtained from the median rank table. Since a 90% confidence level means a 10% risk level, one-half the risk level is at each extreme.

Failure Order	Life Hours	Median Ranks	5% Ranks	95% Ranks
1	45	10.910	0.851	39.304
2	100	26.445	6.285	58.180
3	170	42.141	15.316	72.866
4	240	57.859	27.134	84.684
5	340	73.555	41.820	93.715
6	530	89.090	60.696	99.149

The data is plotted in Figure 9.12. The confidence limits on the MTBF

Figure 9.11 Weibull Plot of Test Data

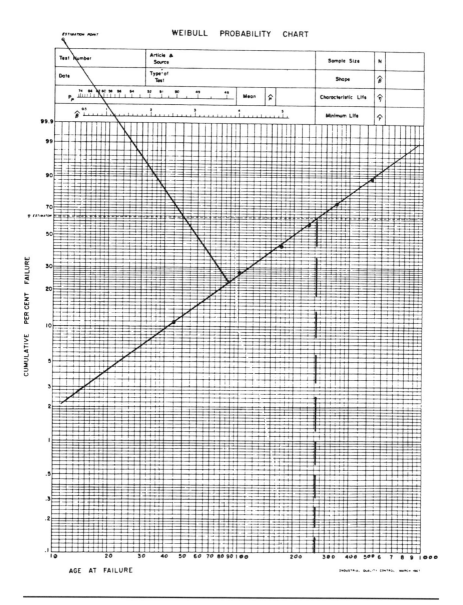

Figure 9.12 Weibull Plot of Confidence Limits

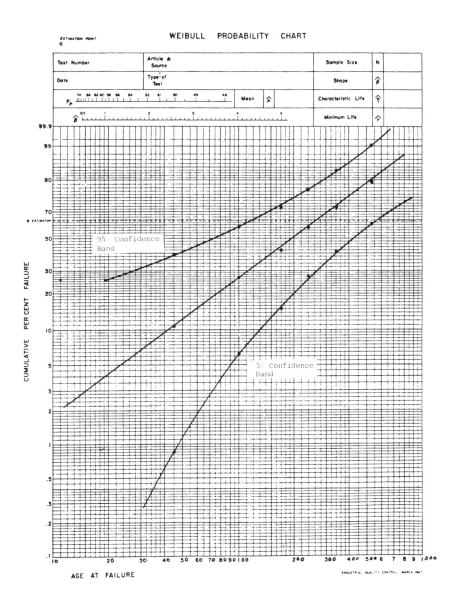

AGE AT FAILURE

are obtained by noting the intersection points of the 63.2% line and the 5% and 95% confidence bands. In this case, $m_{l2} = 110$ hours and $m_{u2} = 560$ hours.

If the 95% confidence band were desired, the 2.5% and 97.5% ranks would have been used.

9.4.3.3 The Shape of Weibull Plots

The type of plot obtained contains much valuable information on the test data. The shape parameter (β) value and the shape of the curve are very important.

On some Weibull papers, a perpendicular line is drawn from the plot to a point on the paper, called the estimation point. This perpendicular line passes through a scale that indicates a β value. On other papers, a line parallel to the plot is drawn through a scale to give the β value.

When $\beta = 1$, the failure rate is constant and the test units are in their useful life period. Where $\beta < 1$, the failure rate is decreasing with time (early life period). When $\beta > 1$, the failure rate increases with time (wearout period). In reality, the unit may be in its useful life period and indicate a β value slightly above or below 1.

Weibull plots may be of two types:

> Linear
> Curved.

Linear plots (Figure 9.13) indicate a single failure mode. The plot is used to determine the MTBF as well as the percentage of units that have failed at a particular time or number of cycles of operation. This is done by drawing a vertical line from the desired value on the x-axis to the plot and then determining the corresponding intersectional point on the y-axis.

Curved plots (Figure 9.14) are indicative of multiple failure modes. The curved plot can usually be separated into its component linear plots by fitting lines parallel to the curved portions. Once linear plots are obtained from the curved plot, information as noted in the previous paragraph can be obtained.

9.4.3.4 The Sudden Death Test

Sudden death testing consists of dividing the test sample into equal groups of samples. Each group is tested until the first failure occurs in the group. At that time, all members of the group are taken off the test. Once all groups have failed, each group is considered as one failure. The

Figure 9.13 Weibull Linear Plot

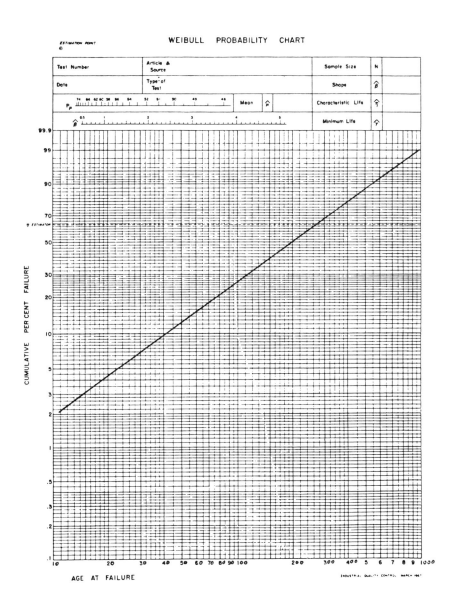

Figure 9.14 Weibull Curved Plot

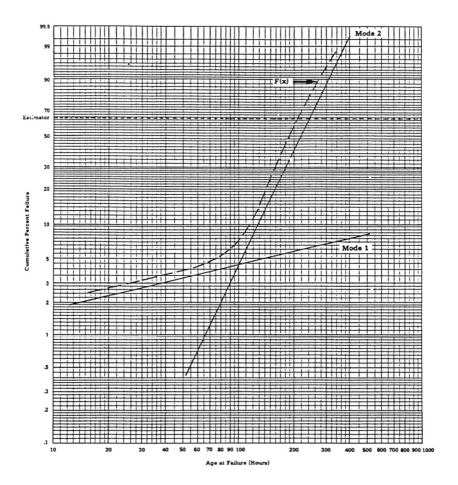

Age at Failure (Hours)

data is plotted on Weibull paper as above. This produces the sudden death line that represents the distribution of lines at the median rank for the first failure.

The median rank for the first failure for N = the number of samples in a group is determined. A horizontal line is drawn from this point on the y-axis and intersects a vertical line drawn from the sudden death line at the 50% level. A line parallel to the sudden death line is drawn at the intersection of these two lines. This is the population line that represents the distribution for all units in the test sample.

Example 9.7

Forty power supplies are to be tested. Randomly divide the power supplies into five groups of eight pumps each. Put all pumps on test in each group simultaneously. The testing proceeds until any pump in each group fails, at which time the testing of all pumps in that group stops. For our example,

Group	Unit Number	Time of Failure hours
1	4	235
2	8	315
3	3	120
4	6	85
5	2	450

To analyze the data, first arrange the failures in ascending hours to failure. The median ranks are determined from the median rank tables in Appendix 2 based on a sample size of N = 5, since there were only five failures.

Failure Order Number	Life in Hours	Median Ranks (%)
1	85	12.95
2	120	31.38
3	235	50.00
4	315	68.62
5	450	87.06

The results are plotted on Weibull paper (Figure 9.15). The resulting line is called the sudden death line. It represents the cumulative distribution of the first failure in eight of the population of power supplies.

The median rank for the first failure in N = 8 is 8.30%, found by looking in the median rank table under N = 8 and Order Number = 1. Thus the sudden death line represents the distribution of the lines

Figure 9.15 Sudden Death Line

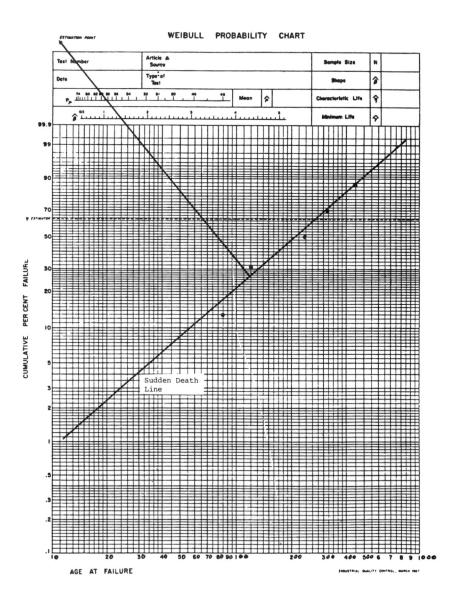

Figure 9.16 Population Line

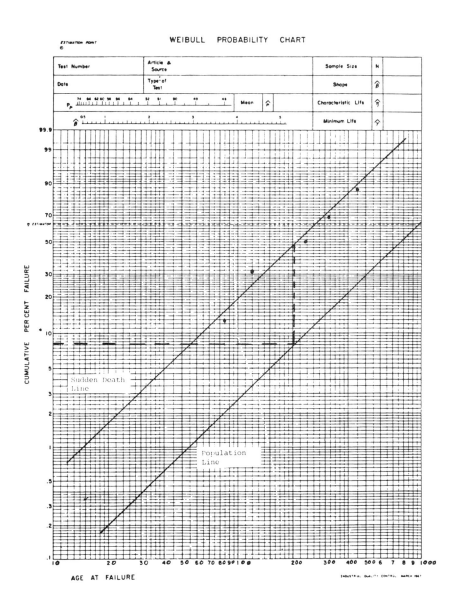

at which 8.3% of the samples are most likely to fail.

To find the population line, draw a vertical line through the intersection of the sudden death line and the horizontal line at the 50% level. Then draw a horizontal line from the 8.3% point on the y-axis until it meets this vertical line. This point is the 8.3% life point of the population. Next, draw a straight line through this point, parallel to the sudden death line, thus determining the population line (Figure 9.16). The MTBF of the population line can be determined by drawing a vertical line from the intersection of the population line and the 63.2% level and reading the corresponding life in hours. In this case, MTBF = 950 hours.

Obtain the confidence limits on this result by choosing the confidence level, e.g., 90%, obtaining the corresponding ranks from the median rank table, e.g., N = 5, 5% rank and 95% rank, and plotting these to obtain the sudden death band lines. Then shift these bands vertically down by a distance equal to the vertical distance between the sudden death line and the population line. These new bands are the exact population confidence bands.

Failure Order	Life Hours	Median Ranks (%)	5% Rank	95% Rank
1	85	12.95	1.02	45.07
2	120	31.38	7.64	65.74
3	235	50.00	18.93	81.07
4	315	68.62	34.26	92.36
5	450	87.06	54.93	98.98

The bands are plotted in Figure 9.17.

9.5 Summary

Hardware validation consists of various types of testing to assure the hardware will operate in its specified environment. Testing is conducted not only in the anticipated environment, but in the worst case environment as well. Tests are conducted on components to verify their reliability in the particular application and to develop reliability parameters for that application.Testing can be conducted in the typical environment or be accelerated where test time is limited. Test results need to be analyzed and presented in a form that is most meaningful to Product Development personnel and management. This may take the form of spread sheets, graphs or pareto analysis.

Parallel with the validation of the hardware, the software must also be validated. This is discussed in the next chapter.

Figure 9.17 Confidence Bands

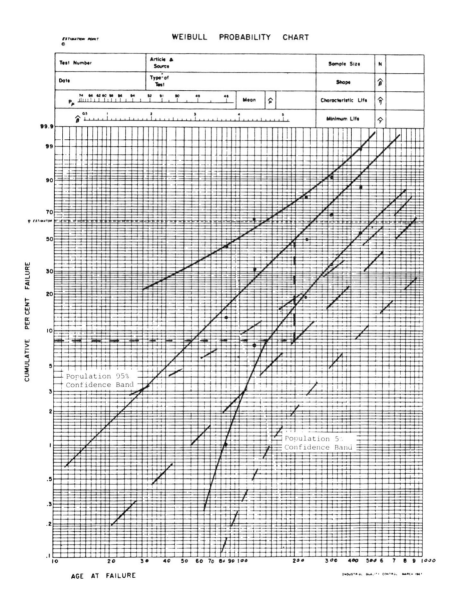

9.6 References

1. Frankel, E. G., *Systems Reliability and Risk Analysis*. The Hague Martinus Nijhoff Publishers, 1984.

2. Kececioglu, D., "Lecture Notes of AME 518 - Reliability Testing," University of Arizona, 1984.

3. Lloyd, D. K. and M. Lipow, *Reliability Management, Methods and Mathematics*. 2nd Edition Milwaukee, Wisconsin: The American Society for Quality Control, 1984.

4. O'Connor, P. D. T., *Practical Reliablity Engineering*. New York: John Wiley and Sons, 1984.

10

The Validation Phase – Software

Once the software program is written, it must be verified and validated to assure it is safe, effective, reliable and satisfies its software specification. Documented evidence of this phase assures control of the phase and satisfies FDA requirements.

"Software verification" is the process of determining whether or not the products of a design phase of the development process fulfill the requirements established during the feasibility phase.

"Software validation" is the process of evaluating software at the end of the software development process to assure compliance with software requirements.

10.1 Software Testing

When testing a software program, it is desirable to add some value to the program. Adding value means raising the quality or reliability of the program. Raising the reliability means finding and removing errors. Thus a program should not be tested to show that it works. Rather, it should be assumed that the program contains errors and the test should find as many errors as possible. This leads to the definition of software testing:

> the process of executing a program with the intent of finding errors.

This differs from the common definition of software testing, which states that testing is the process of demonstrating that a device or module does what is has been specified to do. However, a program that does what it is supposed to do can still contain errors. These errors may appear only when a certain value is handled or when a rarely used branch of the program is executed. A test that is executed to detect errors is a successful one in improving the reliability of the device.

If we assume this definition is a good one, the next question is whether it is practical or even possible to detect all of the errors in a program, especially a program that consists of several million lines of code. In general, it is not. This has implications on the economics of testing, the assumptions the tester will make about the program and the manner in which the test is designed.

10.2 Test Principles

To assist in designing the most successful test and detecting the most errors, a set of guidelines or principles that may appear to be intuitively obvious are often overlooked:

> The test must include a definition of the expected output or result.

> The results of each test must be thoroughly analyzed.

> Tests must be written for invalid and unexpected, as well as valid and expected, input conditions.

> A program must be tested not only to show whether it does what it is supposed to do, but also whether it does what it is not supposed to do.

> The probability of the existence of more errors in a program is proportional to the number of errors already found.

Testing is an extremely creative and intellectually challenging task. This phase of the development process consists of three basic stages:

> Verification and Validation Plan

> Verification and Validation Activity

> Verification and Validation Summary Report.

10.3 Verification and Validation Plan

The first step in the validation process is the formulation of a test plan. This plan outlines the activities to be accomplished in assuring the software package meets its specification. It is a detailed statement of the testing methods used, including:

> Test strategies

> Test completion criteria

Failure definition

Performance range over which the testing and analysis will be performed

Safety analysis

Anticipated use and misuse testing.

The test plan should contain a check sheet for each test and a space for the test personnel to initial when the test is complete.

10.3.1 Test Strategies

Testing strategies are divided into two types:

Black box testing

White box testing.

10.3.1.1 Black Box Testing

Black box testing is a data driven testing scheme. The tester views the program as a black box, that is, the tester is not concerned about the internal behavior and structure of the program. The tester is only interested in finding circumstances in which the program does not behave according to its specifications. Black box testing, used to detect errors, leads to exhaustive input testing, where every possible input condition is a test case.

10.3.1.2 White Box Testing

White box testing is a logic driven testing scheme. The tester examines the internal structure of the program and derives test data from an examination of the program logic. White box testing is concerned with the degree to which test cases exercise or cover the logic of the program. The ultimate white box test is an exhaustive path testing.

10.3.2 Test Completion Criteria

One of the most difficult questions to answer when testing a program is when does the testing end. Some of the more common criteria include:

When the scheduled test time expires

When all test cases execute without detecting errors.

Both criteria are independent of the quality of the program.

More useful criteria include basing test completion on:

    The use of specific test-case-design methodologies

    The detection of a certain number of errors

    The slope of the curve of the plot of the cumulative errors versus cumulative running time approaches zero.

10.3.3 Failure Definition

A software failure may be defined as:

    A departure of the external results of a program operation from program requirements.

A failure must be defined for each software program, based upon its specification, intended application and anticipated environment. Two main types of failures are defined:

    Hard failure

    Soft failure.

10.3.3.1 Hard Failure

A hard failure is one in which the operation of the device is affected to such an extent that rebooting the system does not eliminate the failure.

10.3.3.2 Soft Failure

A soft failure is eliminated by rebooting the system.

10.4 Verification and Validation Activity

Verification and validation activity consists of various levels of software testing to assure the software meets its specification. Such activity consists of:

    Failure Mode Analysis

    Structured Software Testing

    Test data for reliability calculations.

10.4.1 Failure Mode Analysis

Failure mode analysis can be conducted before one byte of code is keyed, if a flow chart, data diagram or similar chart of the program has been developed. The analysis consists of walking through the flow chart or data diagram, testing all possible conditions, especially at decision points and determining the effect on the program. The purpose of the analysis is to determine failure-prone areas and to highlight areas where all possible conditions have not been addressed. By conducting this analysis early in the validation phase, failure prone areas can be addressed without having to rewrite large sections of code.

10.4.2 Structured Software Testing

Software testing should be structured such that all areas, or as many as possible within the program, are exercised and checked for the probability of failure. One successful method in completing this procedure is to begin testing at the lowest level and working to higher, more complex levels. This structured approach consists of:

> Component Testing
> Integration Testing
> System Testing
> Acceptance Testing.

10.4.2.1 Component Testing

Component testing consists of verifying the design and implementation of the specification at the smallest portions of the program, such as the modules and subelements. The test consists of running each module to assure it works and simultaneously inserting errors, possibly through use of an emulator. The test is basically an interface between the programmer and the software environment.

10.4.2.2 Integration Testing

After the modules or subelements have been satisfactorily tested, the next step is to integrate the various modules to assure they can work together.

10.4.2.3 System Testing

The software program is now ready to be tested as a whole to verify the program's compliance with the system objectives. The testing consists of verifying the external software interfaces, assuring the system requirements and assuring the system, as a whole, is operational.

10.4.2.4 Acceptance Testing

To fully accept the software program, the software must be tested in conjunction with the hardware. The next chapter, on device validation, details acceptance testing.

10.4.3 Test Data for Reliability Calculations

During validation activity, software personnel should record each failure when it occurs and the length of time the software ran until it failed. The MTBF can then be calculated as:

$$MTBF = t/r$$

where

t = cumulative running time

r = total number of failures noted

In addition, by recording cumulative errors and plotting them against the cumulative running time, the time when the number of remaining errors is small can be determined. This occurs when the slope of the curve approaches zero.

10.5 Verification and Validation Report

The verification and validation report summarizes the results of the verification and validation activity. The summary contains:

Description of the tasks performed
Time or number of cycles each activity was run
Summary of task results
Summary of errors found and their resolution
Assessment of the software reliability.

In summarizing the errors found, include:

Description and location
Impact
Criticality
Rationale for resolution
Results of retest.

Any deviations from the test plan must be explicitly identified and justified in the test summary.

10.6 Validation Software Review

A software review should be held following completion of the Validation Phase. The review should include:

The final software specification
The validation summary report
The reliability calculations
Any changes since the last review.

The review should be documented and the report made part of the product file.

10.7 Summary

Software testing can be of two types, a test that proves the software does what it has been specified to do and a test that tries to make the software fail so errors can be found. No matter which type is chosen, the validation of a software program is a challenging task. Software has many paths that need to be tested. The difficulty is know when the software has been sufficiently tested.

Validation activity must be sufficient to give the designer confidence that the software operates according to specification and the majority of errors have been removed. To do this, a validation protocol is developed and followed. The testing is conducted in increasingly more complex modes, starting with module testing and ending with system testing. Test results are documented and made part of the product file.

The software and hardware have now been validated. The next chapter discusses the validation of the device.

10.8 References

1. Boehm, B. W., "Software Engineering," *IEEE Transactions on Computers*. Volume C-25, Number 12, December, 1976.

2. Copi, I. M., *Introduction to Logic*. New York: Macmillan, 1968.

3. Dunn, R., *Software Defect Removal*. New York: McGraw-Hill Book Company, 1984.

4. IEEE Standard 1012, *IEEE Standard for Software Verification*

and Validation Plans. New York: Institute of Electrical and Electronic Engineers, 1986.

5. Kahan, J. S., "Validating Computer Systems," *Medical Diagnostic and Device Industry*. March, 1987.

6. Myers, G. T., *The Art of Software Testing*. New York: John Wiley and Sons, 1979.

7. Nesbit, R. A., *Realistic Software Testing and Validation*. Brea, California, Beckman Instruments Diagnostic Systems Group, 1987.

11

The Validation Phase – The Device

The hardware has been tested as an entity, as has the software. The only remaining task to be performed is to verify the hardware and software work together as a system. This formidable task consists of:

Hardware/software compatibility

Environmental testing

Safety analysis

Beta evaluation

Reliability demonstration.

11.1 Hardware/Software Compatibility

During hardware evaluation, components were evaluated for their specific application within the device. Testing showed the hardware works as specified. Software validation proceeded from the module level to module integration, with error introduction included. The software works as specified. The question remains, will the hardware and software work together?

In the Design Phase, a specification was written which detailed the method of hardware/software interaction. To validate this interaction, several tests can be used to verify the success of the specification. The device should be run at the worst case enviroment. This will indicate if stress on the hardware components will affect the software. The voltage should be varied to plus and minus fifteen percent of the specified input voltage. Changes in voltage may affect software. Harmonics of the input voltage may effect software and should be tested. Brownouts should be simulated, by dropping a predetermined number of cycles from the input. Single point failure introduction, through a Failure Mode and Effects Analysis program (see Chapter 9) will yield useful information.

In all cases where failures occur, the cause of the failure, either hardware or software, must be determined and corrected.

11.2 Environmental Testing

Environmental testing is conducted on a device to assure its ability to withstand the environmental stresses associated with its shipping and operational life. Testing is usually conducted on the first devices built in the Manuafcturing area under Manufacturing processes. Environmental testing includes:

> Operating temperature
> Storage temperature
> Thermal shock
> Humidity
> Mechanical shock
> Mechanical vibration
> Impact
> Electrostatic discharge
> Electromagnetic compatibility.

Prior to each test, the device is tested electrically and mechanically to assure it is functioning according to specification. At the conclusion of each environmental test, the device is again tested electrcally and mechanically to determine if the enviromental test has affected the specified operation. Any observed failures will be fixed and a decision to re-run the test made, based on the type of change made and the inherent risk.

11.2.1 Operating Temperature Testing

The operating temperature test assures the device will operate according to specification at the extremes of the typical operating temperature range. The test also analyzes the internal temperatures of the device to assure none exceed the temperature limits of any components.

After the functional checkout, the device has thermocouples placed inside at locations that are predicted to be the hottest. The device is turned ON and placed in a temperature chamber for 4 hours at each of the operating temperature limits as specified in the Product Specification or if no limits are specified, at 0 degrees Centigrade and +55 degrees Centigrade. After testing at the first temperature, the device should be removed from the chamber until the chamber has reached the second temperature. The device is them returned to the chamber for the next 4 hours. Thermocouple readings are recorded continuously on a chart recorder throughout each four hour test period. Where a chart recorder is not available, the readings should be taken every 30 minutes.

The unit is functionally tested after the final temperature exposure. The thermocouple readings are evaluated with regard to the upper extreme of component temperatures.

11.2.2 Storage Temperature Testing

The storage temperature test assures the device will withstand the stresses of the shipping and storage environment.

After the functional checkout, the device is turned OFF and placed in a temperature chamber for eight hours at each of the storage temperature limits as specified in the Product Specification or at −40 degrees Centigrade and +65 degrees Centigrade if no limits are specified. Following each temperature exposure, the device should be removed from the chamber, allowed to come to room temperature and then functionally tested.

11.2.3 Thermal Shock Testing

The thermal shock test assures the device will withstand the stresses of alternate exposure to hot and cold temperatures.

After the functional checkout, the device is turned OFF and placed in a thermal shock chamber with one chamber set at −20 degrees centigrade, the second chamber set at +55 degrees centigrade and the transition time between chambers set at less than five minutes. The minimum time spent at each temperature is one hour. The device should be cycled through a minimum of five cycles of temperature extremes.

The unit is functionally tested after the total number of cycles is completed.

11.2.4 Humidity Testing

The humidity test assures the device will withstand the stresses of exposure to a humid environment.

After the functional checkout, the device is turned off and placed in a humidity chamber with the environment set to 40 degrees Centigrade and 95% relative humidity. The chamber and accessories are so constructed that condensate will not drip on the device. The chamber shall also be transvented to the atmosphere to prevent the buildup of total pressure. The device will be exposed for a minimum of 7 days and a maximum of 21 days.

The unit is allowed to dry following exposure. It is then opened and examined for moisture damage. All observations are documented with photographs if possible. The unit is then functionally tested.

Figure 11.1 Mechanical Shock Parameters

Device		Effective Free Fall Drop Height	Typical Values	
Weight	Greatest Dimension		Acceler-ation	Pulse Duration
(lbs)	(inches)	(inches)	(Gs)	(msec)
< 100	< 36	48	500	2
	> 36	30	400	2
100 - 200	< 36	30	400	2
	> 36	24	350	2
200 - 1000	< 36	24	350	2
	36 - 60	36	430	2
	> 60	24	350	2
> 1000		18	300	2

11.2.5 Mechanical Shock Testing

The mechanical shock test assures the device is able to withstand stresses of handling, shipping and everyday use.

Devices may be tested in the packaged or unpackaged state. Devices may also be tested on a shock table where parameters are set such as in Figure 11.1, to meet the anticipated environment. When using the shock table, several types of waveforms are ordinarily available, depending on the type of impact expected. The haversine waveform simulates impact with a rebound while a sawtooth waveform simulates impact with no rebound. The device may also be dropped the designated distance, from Figure 11.1, on to a hard surface by measuring the height above the floor and dropping the device. One disadvantage of the drop test is the inability to adjust the shock pulse to match the surface and the rebound. With either type of test, the device is normally shocked a maximum of three times in each axis.

Following testing, the device is examined for any internal damage and functionally tested.

11.2.6 Mechanical Vibration Testing

The mechanical vibration test assures the device is able to withstand the vibration stresses of handling, shipping and everyday use, especially where the device is mobile.

Devices may be tested in the packaged or unpackaged state. Packaged vibration testing simulates the evironment the device will experience during shipping. Unpackaged testing simulates the environment the device will experience in everyday use. In the unpackaged state, holes are cut in the device for observation of the internal hardware with a strobe light or for insertion of accelerometers for measuring vibration. Accelerometers are attached to the desired components and their frequencies and amplitudes recorded on an X-Y plotter.

Vibrate the device via a frequency sweep or via random vibration. The random vibration more closely simulates the actual field enviroment, although resonant frequencies and the frequencies of component damage are more easily obtained with the frequency sweep.

When using the frequency sweep, the sweep should be in accordance with the parameters listed in Figure 11.2. Subject the device to three sweeps in one axis at a sweep rate of 0.5 octave/minute. An octave is defined as the interval of two frequencies having a basic ratio of 2. During the sweeps, the acceleration, as listed in Figure 11.2, is the maximum acceleration observed at any point on the device.

Figure 11.2 Mechanical Vibration Parameters

Locale	Format	Frequency Sweep	Acceleration
Domestic	Unpackaged	5 - 200 - 5 Hz	1.5 G
International	Unpackaged	5 - 300 - 5 Hz	2.0 G
Domestic	Packaged	5 - 300 - 5 Hz	1.5 G
International	Packaged	5 - 500 - 5 Hz	2.0 G

Resonant frequencies are determined either through accelerometer readings or through observation of the internal hardware. Resonances are defined as board or component movement of a minimum of twice the difference between the device and table acceleration. Severe resonance is usually accompanied by a steady drone from the resonating component. Once resonant frequencies are determined, a dwell at each resonant frequency for 15 minutes follows the frequency sweeps.

The above tests are repeated until all three orthogonal axes have been tested. The unit is examined for physical damage and functionally tested after each axis is completed.

11.2.7 Impact Testing

Impact testing assures the ability of the device to withstand the collision stresses of shipping and for mobile devices the everyday use environment. The test simulates large, mobile devices bumping into walls or door frames while being moved.

The test is conducted by rolling a device down an inclined ramp and allowing it to slam into a solid wall or by attaching the device to an ad-

justable piston drive, which is set to slam the device into a solid wall
with a predetermined force.
The unit is functionally tested following impact.

11.2.8 Electrostatic Discharge

Electrostatic discharge testing assures the ability of the device to withstand short duration voltage transients caused by static electricity, capacitive
or inductive effects and load switching. For software-controlled devices,
a differentiation between hard failures, that is, failures that cause the
device to become inoperable and not rebootable and soft failures, that is,
failures that cause the device to become inoperable but rebootable, must
be made and the acceptability of each defined, according to risk.
The device is placed on a grounded metal plane. Static discharges
are delivered to the four quadrants of the plane and to appropriate places
on the device, such as front panel, back panel, keyboard, etc., from a
static generator or a current injector. One-shot static charges should be
delivered directly to the device and to the air surrounding the device.
Where the device is connected to accessory equipment via cables, such
as analog or RS-232 cables, static discharges should be delivered in the
area of the cable connections, on both pieces of equipment. All discharges
should be one-shot and should begin at 2,000 volts and increase in 2,000
volt increments until the maximum of 20,000 volts is reached.
The unit is functionally tested following application of electrostatic
discharge.

11.2.9 Electromagnetic Compatibility

Electromagnetic Compatiblity (EMC) testing is conducted to determine
the maximum levels of electromagnetic emissions the device is allowed
to produce and to determine the minimum levels electromagnetic interference to which the device must not be susceptible. Medical devices,
especially those used in the Operating Room environment, must not in-
terfere with the operation of other devices or have its operation inter-
fered with by other devices through electromagnetic radiations.
It is particularly important to conduct EMC testing on products containing:

Digital circuitry, especially microprocessor-based devices

Circuits containing clock or crystal oscillators

Devices where data information is transmitted via a telemet-
ric or radio frequency link.

Monitors, used in close proximity to other devices or where they cause feedback to other devices.

Tests should be conducted in a testing laboratory containing an anechoic chamber or shielded chamber of sufficient size to adequately contain the test. The device is configured and operated in a manner that approximates its use in a medical facility. When necessary, a dummy load and/or signal simulator may be employed to duplicate actual equipment operation. As of this writing, no comprehensive EMC test for medical devices exists. The test MDS-201-0004, developed by Mc Donnell Douglas in 1979 and adopted as a voluntary standard by the FDA, met the typical hospital environment in 1979, but not today. Some medical groups attempted to produce a standard after a complete review of the current hospital environment, but because of the immensity of this task, they have not completed it. As a result, many companies have developed their own EMC tests, using part of MDS-201-0004 and part of FCC Regulation, Part 15. Failures must be defined when designing the test.

It is a known that most Bovie units, especially older ones, produce radiation that is worse than that called out in any standard. Thus, as a practical approach to EMC, many companies use a Bovie unit in the vicinity of the test device to check its susceptibility. In the laboratory environment, the test device can be used in the presence of other devices to test its radiation.

Subject all devices to conducted and radiated emissions and to conducted and radiated susceptibility testing. Monitor the functionality of the unit throughout the test.

11.3 Safety Analysis

Conduct safety analysis to assure the device is safe and effective for its intended use. The device must not cause a hazard to the user or the patient.

Due to the variety of medical devices with many degrees of complexity, the following should be included in the safety analysis program:

Safety review personnel must have a thorough understanding of the operation of the device. Personnel should review pertinent documentation, such as drawings, test reports and manuals prior to the analysis.

Make a representative device available for the review. It will be subject to disassembly.

Use a checklist especially prepared for the paricular device for the analysis.

Address each area of concern immediately. Safety release is not granted until the device has no apparent areas of concern

Safety release the device via a release letter only after all areas of concern are addressed.

Retain the checklist and release letter as part of the Product file.

Specifically prepare a comprehensive checklist for the device under analysis. Areas to be addressed in the checklist include, but are not limited to:

Voltages
Operating frequencies
Leakage currents
Dielectric withstand
Environmental specifications
Grounding impedance
Power cord and plug
Electrical insulation
Abnormal operations
Physical stability
Corrosion protection
Circuit breakers and fuses
Color coding
Ergonomic specifications
Standards Conformance
Alarms, warnings and indicators
Mechanical design integrity.

The checklist should be signed by the analyst(s) after completion of the analysis. Figure 11.3 shows an example of one page of such a checklist.

11.4 Beta Evaluation

Beta evaluation or clinical trials are the first opportunity to test the device in its intended application. Beta evaluation determines if the device actually fills the customer's expectations and the need in the marketplace. It helps determine the future success the device or the lack of it.

Any Beta evaluation should be governed by a Beta contract between the device manufacturer and the Beta site. This contract outlines the specifics of the testing and details the requirements and expectations of both parties.

Figure 11.3 Safety Analysis Checklist

Characteristic	Comment
Operating Voltage	
Maximum Wattage	
Leakage Current	
Dielectric Withstand	
Power Plug Rating	
Strain Relief	
Grounding	
Physical Stability	
Circuit Breakers	
Alarms	
Color Coding	

In many ways, Beta evaluation is a more severe test of the device than any test carried out in the laboratory. There is not only the user learning curve to be experienced, but also the typical user misuse to which the device will be routinely subjected. It is the first chance to develop a MTBF value for the device based on actual usage. By use of a hour meter in the device, which will record the actual operation time, an accurate MTBF value can be calculated that can then be compared to those values determined from laboratory testing. These may be an indication of the effectiveness of the laboratory tests.

The units used in Beta evaluation are either Engineering prototypes or the first units built under Manufacturing processes. The units must be safety tested prior to being sent to the Beta site.

All failures experienced at the Beta site should be documented as to:

> Time of failure
> Observation
> Mode of failure
> Failure mechanism.

Failure data is then analyzed to determine reliability parameters and detect failure trends.

Use the times of failures to calculate values of MTBF. By plotting all early failures by time of failure, a pattern of infant mortality failures may be determined, which may cause the suggested burn-in scheme for the device to be adjusted. The failure analysis is also used to solidify anticipated warranty expenses.

Upon completion of the evaluation, the Beta site should write a summary report detailing the test procedures, test results, any corrective action and its result. Any deviations from the approved protocol must be explicitly identified and justified.

11.5 Reliability Demonstration

Reliability demonstration, or life testing, is the culmination of all other product development activities. For the first time, the final product, as the customer will receive it, is available and can be tested for the actual MTBF value. As the majority of the problems should have been eliminated earlier in the development process, this test should basically be a failure-free run to a MTBF value.

The units tested are the first built under Manufacturing processes following product release. They contain the final version of hardware and software and have been burned-in according to Manufacturing procedures.

The units should be kept in an area with a constantly controlled environment, where temperature and humidity are monitored. The temperature and humidity should be set to values typically seen in the field.

The test should consist of operating the units as they would be in normal use. The units operate 24 hours per day. Appropriate inputs from accessory equipment is employed. Device outputs are monitored and documented.

Testing continues until the desired MTBF value has been achieved at a 95% confidence level. Test results are summarized in a final test report.

11.6 Summary

Device testing is the final step in the validation phase. It is the culmination of all previous testing as the hardware and the software begin to interact. The testing attempts to look at the enviroment the device will experience in actual use. Therefore, testing includes environmental, safety, clinical and long term reliability demonstration.

Once the testing is completed, the data must be analyzed to indicate how safe, effective and reliable the device really is. Data analysis is discussed in the next chapter.

11.7 References

1. ASTM, *Annual Book of ASTM Standards*. Philadelphia: American Society for Testing Materials, 1975.

2. Canadian Standards Association, *Standard 22.2*. Rexdale, Ontario: Canadian Standards Association.

3. Frankel, E. G., *Systems Reliability and Risk Analysis*. The Hague: Martinus Nijhoff Publishers, 1984.

4. IEC, *Standard 601.1*. Geneva, Switzerland: Bureauaa Central de la Commission Electrotechnique Internationale.

5. Kececioglu, D., "Lecture Notes of AME-518 - Reliability Testing," The University of Arizona, 1984.

6. Lloyd, D. K. and M. Lipow, *Reliability Management, Methods and Mathematics*. 2nd Edition Milwaukee, Wisconsin: American Society for Quality Control, 1984.

7. MIL-HDBK-108, *Sampling Procedure and Tables for Life and Reliability Testing*. Washington, DC: Department of Defense, 1960.

8. MIL-STD-781, Reliability Qualification and Production Approval Tests. Washington, DC: Department of Defense, 1977.

9. MIL-STD-810, *Environmental Test Methods*. Washington, DC: Department of Defense, 1978.

10. MIL-STD-1635, *Reliability Growth Testing*. Washington, DC: Department of Defense, 1978.

11. O'Connor, P. D. T., *Practical Reliability Engineering*. New York: John Wiley and Sons, 1984.

12. Reliability Analysis Center, *Reliability Design Handbook*. Chicago: ITT Research Institute, 1976.

12

The Validation Phase – Data Analysis

The heart of reliability is the analysis of data from which desired reliability parameters can be calculated. These parameters are calculated from testing throughout the product development process. Early calculations are updated as the program progresses and the presence or lack of reliability improvement becomes apparent.

Reliability parameter calculation assumes the product is in the useful life period of the bathtub curve. During this period, the failure rate is constant and the exponential distribution is used for calculations. In standards and handbooks where failure rates and MTBF values are listed, the same assumption is made and the exponential distribution is used.

Calculations of some parameters, such as MTBF, depend upon the termination mode of the test. Time terminated tests, where tests are ended after a predetermined time period has elapsed, are calculated in a manner different from failure terminated tests, where tests are ended after a predetermined number of units have failed.

Following is a review of the calculations necessary to determine:

> Failure rate
> MTBF
> Reliability
> Confidence limits.

In addition, graphical analysis and its application to reliability data are discussed.

12.1 Failure Rate

Failure rate is the number of failures per million hours of operation. For devices in their useful life period, the failure rate is the reciprocal of the MTBF. When calculating the reciprocal, the failure rate must be in failures per hour.

Example 12.1

An EEG machine has a MTBF of 4380 hours. What is the failure rate?

$$\lambda = 1/MTBF$$

$$= 1/4380$$

$$= 0.000228 \text{ failures per hour}$$

$$= 228 \text{ failures per million hours}$$

Example 12.2

Ten power supplies are put on test, to be terminated after each has completed 1000 hours of operation. Two power supplies fail, one at 420 hours and the other at 665 hours. What is the failure rate of the power supplies?

Eight units completed 1000 hours.

$$\text{Total test time} = 8(1000) + 420 + 665$$

$$= 9085 \text{ hours}$$

$$\text{Failure rate} = \text{number of failures/total test time}$$

$$= 2/9085$$

$$= 0.000220 \text{ failures per hour}$$

$$= 220 \text{ failures per million hours}$$

12.2 Mean Time Between Failures (MTBF)

Mean Time Between Failures is the time at which 63% of the operational devices in the field will have failed. MTBF is the reciprocal of the failure rate. It is also calculated from test data dependent upon the type of test run, e.g., time terminated or failure terminated, and upon whether the failed units were replaced or not. Five different methods of MTBF calculation are available:

Time terminated, failed parts replaced

Time terminated, no replacement

Failure terminated, failed parts replaced

Failure terminated, no replacement

No failures observed during the test.

12.2.1 Time Terminated, Failed Parts Replaced

MTBF = N(td)/r

where

N = number of units tested

td = test duration

r = number of failures

Example 12.3

The performance of ten pressure monitors is monitored while operating for a period of 1200 hours. The test results are listed below. Every failed units is replaced immediately. What is the MTBF?

Unit Number	Time of Failure (hours)
1	650
2	420
3	130 and 725
4	585
5	630 and 950
6	390
7	No Failure
8	880
9	No Failure
10	220 and 675

N = 10

r = 11

td = 1200 hours

MTBF = N(td)/r

= 10(1200)/11

= 1091 hours

12.2.2 Time Terminated, No Replacement

$$\text{MTBF} = (\sum_{i=1}^{r} T_i) + (N-r)\,td/r$$

where

N = number of units tested

td = test duration

r = number of failures

T_i = individual failure times

Example 12.4

The performance of ten oxygen monitors is monitored while operating for a period of 1200 hours. The test results are listed below. Failed units are not replaced. What is the MTBF?

Unit Number	Time of Failure (hours)
1	650
2	420
3	130
4	585
5	630
6	390
7	No Failure
8	880
9	No Failure
10	220

$$\text{MTBF} = (\sum_{i=1}^{r} T_i) + (N-r)\,td/r$$

$$= (650+420+130+585+630+390+880+220) + 2(1200)/8$$

$$= (3905 + 2400)/8$$

$$= 788 \text{ hours}$$

12.2.3 Failure Terminated, Failed Parts Replaced

$$\text{MTBF} = N(td)/r$$

where

N = Number of units tested

td = test duration

r = number of failures

Example 12.5

Six neural stimulators were placed on test until all units failed, the last occurring at 850 hours. The test results are listed below. Every failed unit, except the last one, is replaced immediately. What is the MTBF?

Unit Number	Time of Failure (hours)
1	130
2	850
3	120 and 655
4	440
5	725
6	580

$$\text{MTBF} = N(td)/r$$

$$= 6(850)/7$$

$$= 729 \text{ hours}$$

12.2.4 Failure Terminated, No Replacement

$$\text{MTBF} = (\sum_{i=1}^{r} T_i) + (N-r)\,td/r$$

where

T_i = individual times of failure

N = Number of units tested

td = test duration

r = number of failures

Example 12.6

Six neural stimulators were placed on test until all units failed. The last failure occurred at 850 hours. Failed units were not replaced. Test results are listed below. What is the MTBF?

Unit Number	Time of Failure (hours)
1	130
2	850
3	120
4	440
5	725
6	580

$$\text{MTBF} = (\sum_{i=1}^{r} T_i) + (N-r)\,td/r$$

$$= (130+850+120+440+725+580) + 0(850)/6$$

$$= 3945 + 0/6$$

$$= 658 \text{ hours}$$

12.2.5 No Failures Observed

For the case where no failures are observed, an MTBF value cannot be calculated. A lower one-sided confidence limit must be calculated and the MTBF stated to be greater that that value.

$$m_L = 2(Ta)/\chi^2_{\alpha;2}$$

where

m_L = lower one-sided confidence limit

Ta = total test time

$\chi^2_{\alpha;2}$ = the Chi-Square value from the table in Appendix 1, where α is the risk level and 2 is the degrees of freedom

Example 12.7

Twelve power supplies are tested for 2500 hours without failure. What is the MTBF at a 90% confidence level?

$$N = 12$$

$$td = 2500$$

$$r = 0$$
$$1 - \alpha = 0.90$$
$$\alpha = 0.10$$
$$Ta = N(td) = 12(2500) = 30000$$
$$m_L = 2(Ta)/\chi^2_{\alpha;2r + 2}$$
$$= 2(30000)/\chi_{0.10;2}$$
$$= 60000/4.605$$
$$= 13029 \text{ hours}$$

We can then state, with 90% confidence, that the MTBF is 13029 hours.

12.3 Reliability

Reliability is defined as the probability that an item will perform a required function, under specified conditions, for a specified period of time, at a desired confidence level. Reliability may be calculated from either the failure rate or the MTBF. The resultant number is the percentage of units that will survive the specified time.

Reliability can vary between 0 (no reliability) and 1.0 (perfect reliability). The closer the value is to 1.0, the better the reliability will be.

To calculate the parameter "reliability," two parameters are required:

Either the failure rate or the MTBF

The mission time or specified period of operation

$$\text{Reliability} = \exp(- \lambda t)$$
$$= \exp (- t/\text{MTBF})$$

where

$$\lambda = \text{failure rate}$$
$$t = \text{time}$$
$$\text{MTBF} = \text{Mean Time Between Failure}$$

Example 12.8

Using the data in Example 12.2, calculate the reliability of the power supplies for an operating period of 3200 hours.

$$\lambda = \text{failure rate} = 220 \text{ failures per million hours}$$

for the equation, λ must be in failures per hour thus, $220/1000000 = 0.000220$ failures per hour

$$t = 3200 \text{ hours}$$

$$\text{Reliability} = \exp(- \lambda\, t)$$

$$= \exp\ -(0.000220)(3200)$$

$$= \exp\ -(0.704)$$

$$= 0.495$$

This states that after 3200 hours of operation, one half the power supplies in operation will not have failed.

Example 12.9

Using the time terminated, no replacement case, calculate the reliability of the pressure monitors for 500 hours of operation.

$$\text{Reliability} = \exp\ -(\lambda t)$$

$$= \exp\ -(t/\text{MTBF})$$

$$= \exp\ -(500/788)$$

$$= \exp\ -(0.635)$$

$$= 0.530$$

where

$$t = \text{time of operation}$$

$$\text{MTBF} = \text{mean time between failure for the device}$$

Thus, 53% of the pressure monitors will not fail during the 500 hours of operation.

12.4 Confidence Level

Confidence level is the probability that a given statement is correct. When a 90% confidence level is used, the probability that the findings are valid for the device population is 90%.

Confidence level is designated as:

$$\text{Confidence level} = 1 - \alpha$$

where

$$\alpha = \text{the risk level}$$

Example 12.10

Test sample size is determined using a confidence level of 98%. What is the risk level?

$$\text{Confidence Level} = 1 - \alpha$$
$$\alpha = 1 - \text{confidence level}$$
$$= 1 - 0.98$$
$$= 0.02 \text{ or } 2\%$$

12.5 Confidence Limits

Confidence limits are defined as the extremes of a confidence interval within which the unknown has a designated probability of being included. If the identical test was repeated several times with different samples of a device, it is probable that the MTBF value calculated from each test would not be identical. However, the various values would fall within a range of values about the true MTBF value. The two values which mark athe end points of the range are the lower and upper confidence limits.

Calculation of confidence limits depends on whether the test was time or failure terminated.

12.5.1 Time Terminated Confidence Limits

$$m_L = 2(Ta)/\chi^2_{\alpha/2;2r+2}$$

where

$$m_L = \text{lower confidence limit}$$
$$Ta = \text{total test time}$$
$$\chi^2_{\alpha/2;2r+2} = \text{Chi square value from Appendix 1 for } \alpha/2 \text{ risk level and } 2r+2 \text{ degrees of freedom}$$
$$m_U = 2(Ta)/\chi^2_{1-\alpha/2;2r}$$

Example 12.11

Using the data from the time terminated, no replacement data from Example 12.3, at a 90% confidence limit:

$$Ta = 6305 \text{ hours}$$

$$\alpha = 1 - \text{confidence level} = 0.10$$

$$\alpha/2 = 0.05$$

$$r = 8$$

$$2r+2 = 18$$

$$m_L = 2(6305)/\chi^2_{0.05;18}$$

$$= 12610/28.869$$

$$= 437 \text{ hours}$$

$$m_U = 2(6305)/\chi^2_{0.95;16}$$

$$= 12610/7.962$$

$$= 1584 \text{ hours}$$

Therefore:

$$437 < MTBF < 1584 \text{ hours}$$
or the true MTBF lies between 437 and 1584 hours.

12.5.2 Failure Terminated Confidence Limits

$$m_L = 2(Ta)/\chi^2_{\alpha/2;2r}$$

and

$$m_U = 2(Ta)/\chi^2_{1-\alpha/2;2r}$$

Example 12.12

Using the data from the failure terminated, no replacement data from Example 12.5 at a 95% confidence limit:

$$Ta = 3945 \text{ hours}$$

$$\alpha = 0.05$$

$$\alpha/2 = 0.025$$

$$1 - \alpha/2 = 0.975$$
$$r = 6$$
$$2r = 12$$
$$m_L = 2(3945)/\chi^2_{0.025;12}$$
$$= 7890/23.337$$
$$= 338 \text{ hours}$$
$$m_U = 2(3945)/\chi^2_{0.975;12}$$
$$= 7890/4.404$$
$$= 1792 \text{ hours}$$

Therefore:

$$338 < \text{MTBF} < 1792$$

12.6 Minimum Life

The term "minimum life" of a device is the time of occurrence of the first failure.

12.7 Graphical Analysis

Graphical analysis depicts test data or field information. It can show failure trends, determine when a manufacturing learning curve is nearly complete, indicate the severity of field problems or determine the effect of a burn-in program.

Several type of graphical analysis are advantageous in reliability analysis:

  Pareto Analysis

  Graphical Plotting

  Weibull Analysis.

12.7.1 Pareto Analysis

Pareto analysis is a plot of individual failures versus the frequency of the failures. The individual failures are listed on the x-axis and the frequency of occurrence on the y-axis. The result is a histogram of problems and their severity. The problems are usually plotted with the most frequent on the left. Once the results are obtained, appropriate action can be taken. Figure 12.1 is an example of a pareto analysis based on the following data:

Problem	Frequency
Software Problems	5
Leaks	3
Defective Parts	68
Cable Problems	10
Missing Parts	86
Shipping Damage	60

Figure 12.1 Pareto Analysis

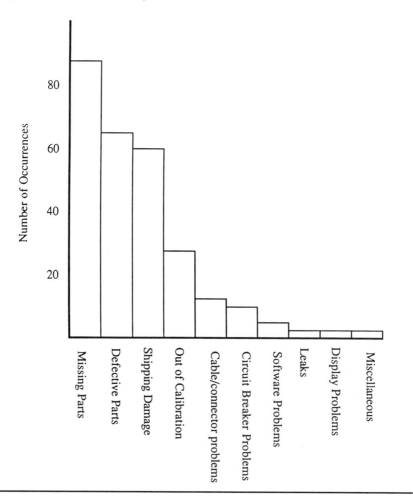

12.7.2 Graphical Plotting

When plotting data, time is usually listed on the x-axis and the parameter to be analyzed on the y-axis.

Example 12.13

Nerve stimulators were subjected to 72 hours of burn-in at ambient temperature prior to shipment to customers. Reports of early failures were grouped into 50 hours intervals and showed the following pattern:

Hourly Increment	Number of Failures
0 - 50	12
51 - 100	7
101 - 150	4
151 - 200	1
201 - 250	1

Figure 12.2 is a plot of the data. The data indicates the number of failures begins to level off at approximately 200 hours. The burn-in was changed to an accelerated burn-in equal to 300 hours of operation.

Figure 12.2 Plot of Field Data

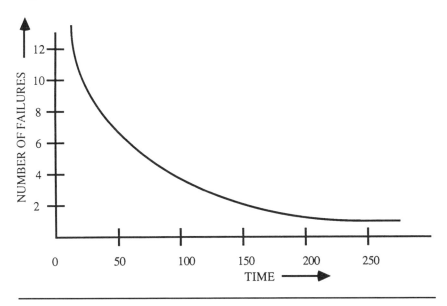

12.7.3 Weibull Plotting

The Weibull distribution was introduced in 1949 by W. Weibull of Sweden as a convenient method of analyzing mechanical fatigue data. Since its introduction, it has been used extensively in areas such as bearing fatigue data and predicition about the failure of automotive parts.

The Weibull distribution has properties which permit it to be fitted to many kinds of data. This results in wide confidence intervals as increased generality results in decreased precision. The distribution used three parameters:

> The scale parameter - alpha
> The shape parameter - beta
> The location parameter - gamma

The scale parameter controls the amount of skewness or spreading from left to right. The shape parameter controls the shape of the distribution function. The location parameter establishes the position of the left end of the distribution and is usually considered to be zero.

The shape parameter (beta) is taken as an indicator of the portion of the life cycle the data represents. When beta is less than one, the data is indicative of the infant mortality period of the product. When beta is equal to one, the data is indicative of the useful life period. When beta is greater than one, the data is indicative of the wearout period of the life cycle.

Weibull paper is a logarithmic plotting paper constructed with the y-axis representing the cumulative probability of failure and the x-axis representing a time value. Data points are established from failure data, with the failure times arranged in increasing order or value of occurrence. Corresponding median ranks are assigned from a percent rank table based on the sample size. The data is plotted and the MTBF is determined at the intersection of the 63.2% point on the y-axis and the plotted curve by dropping a line from this point to the x-axis. Confidence limits can also be determined by this procedure.

Linear plots indicate a single failure mode (Figure 12.3). The plot is used to determine the MTBF as well as the percentage of units that have failed at a particular time or number of cycles of operation. Curved plots are indicative of multiple failure modes (Figure 12.4). The curved plot can be separated into its component linear plots. Once the linear plots are obtained, MTBF and percentage data can be determined for each failure mode.

Details of completing a Weibull plot are discussed beginning with section 9.4.3.1.

Figure 12.3 Linear Weibull Plot

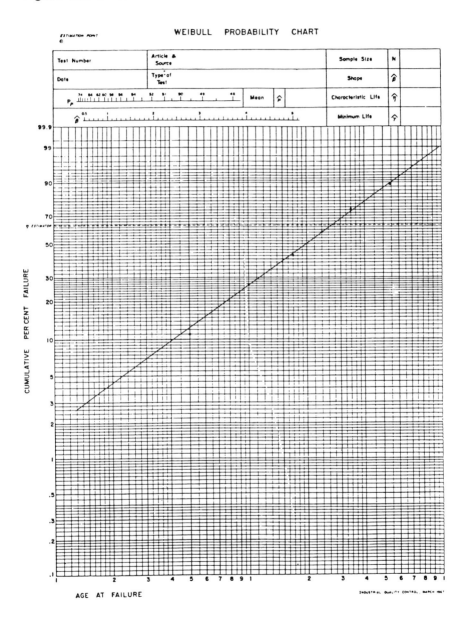

Figure 12.4 Curved Weibull Plot

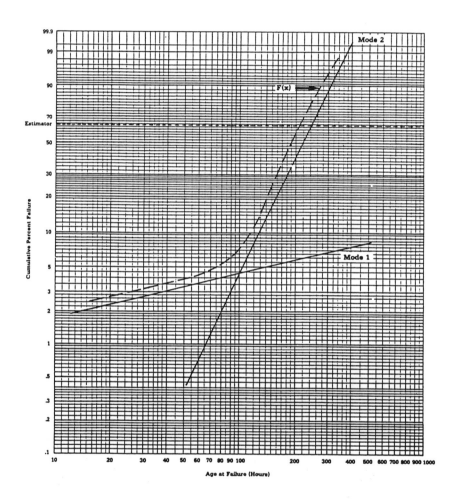

12.8 Summary

Data analysis is the heart of reliability. It gives meaning to the information ovtained from lab tests or field use. The analysis may take the form of parameter calculation or graphical representation of data. The results are used to monitor reliability growth, detect problems or compare one device to another.

Now that the device has been designed, validated and characterized, it is ready to be manufactured.

12.9 References

1. Frankel, E. G., *System Reliability and Risk Analysis*. The Hague: Martinus Nijhoff Publishers, 1984.

2. Kececioglu, D., "Lecture Notes of AME 518 - Reliability Testing," University of Arizona, 1984.

3. King, J. R., *Probability Charts for Decision Making*. New Hampshire: Team, 1971.

4. Lloyd, D. K. and M. Lipow, *Reliability Management, Methods and Mathematics*. 2nd Edition Milwaukee, Wisconsin: The American Society for Quality Control, 1984.

5. Mann, N. R. et al., *Methods for Statistical Analysis of Reliability and Life Data*. New York: John Wiley and Sons, 1974.

6. Nelson, W., *Applied Life Data Analysis*. New York: John Wiley and Sons, 1982.

7. O'Connor, P. D. T., *Practical Reliability Engineering*. New York: John Wiley and Sons, 1984.

13

The Manufacturing Phase

To remain competitive, manufacturers must move from an environment in which product problems are removed by inspection to one in which the process is controlled. Manufacturing excellence can be attained only by designing products and processes to address potential problems before they occur. The Manufacturing phase does not begin when the design is released to production. It began when the device was in the feasibility phase and continued through the design and validation phases.

13.1 Product Release

Product release to production is an integral part of the Product Development process. It is the conclusion of development activity and indicates an acceptable comfort level with the design of the product.

The project team conducts a product release review meeting at the completion or near completion of development activity. All previous development activity is reviewed and action items assigned for any uncompleted activity. Reliability Assurance presents a summary of reliability activity conducted to date. Activity is monitored on a release check sheet, such as that shown in Figure 13.1. Activity is initialed as it is completed. Any activities listed as not completed must be addressed before final release is granted. Any activity indicated as 'waived' will require a rationale in the final summary report. The status of production documentation and parts ordering is discussed and action items assigned.

Product release is categorized into two types:

Conditional

Final.

Figure 13.1 Reliability Release Check Sheet

Activity	Initials
Completion of the Reliability Assurance Test Plan	
Classification of the Device	
Classification of Components and identification of major characteristics	
Completion of the initial reliability hardware prediction	
Completion of drawing and documentation review	
Performance of a FMEA	
Establishment of burn-in requirements	
Approval of the Product Specification	
Addressed domestic and foreign standard requirements	
Submission of Product Approval	
Completion of Safety Review	
Completion of Software Reviews and QA	
Completion of Beta Evaluation	
Completion of Environmental Testing	
Completion of Reliability Demonstration	
Completion of documentation review	

13.1.1 Conditional Release

Conditional release is given when reliability activity has not been completed but no problems exist that have not been resolved. Conditional release is granted such that the final release is contingent on successful completion of the remaining activity. The conditionial release specifically lists all contingencies upon which the final release is dependent.

13.1.2 Final Release

The final product release indicates the completion of all product development activity, including design, testing, parameter calculation and summary reports. It is the indication that reliability goals have been satisfied.

13.2 Structured Manufacturing Process

When a product is subjected to a reliability assurance program in design and is tested to assure reliability, that is no guarantee that the product, as shipped, is reliable. Unless the product is manufactured reliably, the design effort is for naught. Reliability must be in the mind of each individual involved in the manufacturing process. A reliable Manufacturing process is structured to include:

> Design involvement
> Component activity
> Burn-in activity
> Assembly
> Test and inspection
> System burn-in
> Failure analysis
> Statistical process control
> Electrostatic discharge protection.

13.2.1 Design Involvement

Manufacturing involvement early in the design process will assure the production of a design that can be easily manufactured without reliability degradation.

Manufacturing Engineering, an engineering group within manufacturing, develops overall test strategies to assure the most complete fault coverage. They also provide detailed cost information about possible alternatives, so that cost effective component and system burn-in schemes can be selected. They provide guidelines for testability of electronic printed circuit boards and propose alternatives that make the design easier to test.

13.2.2 Component Activity

Initial component activity began during the design phase when components were specified and evaluated for their application in the design, component reliability was reviewed, requirements were established and initial assessment and audits of vendors took place. Orders were placed following the design release meeting. What remains is:

> Establishing incoming requirements
> Qualifying components
> Establishing lot control for the components.

13.2.2.1 Incoming Requirements

A file is established on each component containing:

> Appropriate component drawings
>
> Incoming test specification, if any
>
> Record of incoming history.

Drawings should contain the appropriate dimensions, especially those which are to be verified at incoming. Where off-the-shelf parts are purchased, the requirement may be to assure the part number on the package is correct.

Where testing is to be done at incoming, the test specification must be as detailed as possible. The specification should indicate the type of equipment necessary to conduct the test and the procedure for performing it.

A record of incoming history by component should be kept, either on file or in the computer. The record should contain:

> Component part number
> Vendor(s)
> Delivery date
> Number of components delivered
> Number of components rejected.

These records can be used to produce a history of component deliveries and assist in determining the quality of the vendor.

13.2.2.2 Component Qualification

Products should be manufactured using only qualified components. Components may be qualified for use in a particular product in several ways, depending on the criticality of the device. Components may be subjected to a formal qualification procedure, which may include enviromental and life testing and a review of the history of the vendor and the component. Qualification may consist of reviewing the history of deliveries and rejects. For example, a vendor is qualified after three deliveries with no rejects and continues to be qualified with no rejects. When a delivery contains rejects, the vendor is disqualified and can only be requalified by three consecutive deliveries with no rejects.

13.2.2.3 Lot Control

Once components are accepted at incoming, they should be placed under lot control. This allows problems to be tracked easily, giving the extent of the problem or at least placing it within a range of dates. By storing lots separate from other lots, problem lots can be removed easier. When a First In, First Out (FIFO) system is in effect, it can be accomplished more efficiently with lot control.

13.2.3 Burn-In Activity

Burn-in is defined as the cycling of parts or assemblies, under ambient or accelerated conditions, which simulate the life of the component in its intended application.

The purpose of a burn-in procedure is to detect and eliminate weak components before they are placed in the field. The burn-in process attempts to take each component past its infant mortality period and into its useful life period. Conventional wisdom states that components, which survive past 1000 hours of normal use, have a very low probability of failure until thousands of hours later in life. For this reason, most burn-in procedures are designed to reach the 1000 hour point in the component's life cycle. By accelerating the procedure via high temperature, the burn-in time can be greatly reduced. Care must be taken in establishing high temperature procedures, as higher temperatures accelerate the aging and thus the time to failure of the components.

Several decisions must be made in regard to component burn-in:

Whether to burn-in at all
What components to burn-in
How long to burn-in
What type of burn-in.

13.2.3.1 To Burn-In or Not to Burn-In

Referring to the component classification discussed in Chapter 9:

Level I components, because of their potential safety hazard and the effect of their failure on the system, should be burned-in or purchased as a burned-in component from the vendor.

The requirements for Level II component burn-in are the option of the Product Development team. Since there is no safety concern, the functionality of the component and its effect on the system must be weighed against the cost and lead time of burn-in as well as the cost involved in finding a bad part in the latter stages of development or in the field.

Level III components do not need to be burned-in.

13.2.3.2 Length of Burn-In

The length of the burn-in brings the component out of its infant mortality period and into its useful life period. Where history exists on similar products, the burn-in requirements for those products will assist in determining the requirements for this product. If there were many early field problems, the burn-in time may need to be increased. If there were no early field failures, the burn-in was sufficient.

Where no history exists, a sample burn-in procedure may be tested and the results analyzed. Results will indicate if the length of time is sufficient or not.

13.2.3.3 Types of Burn-In

Two types of burn-in are commonly used. Selection of the appropriate type depends on component use and application:

> Static burn-in applies only power and ground to the parts

> Dynamic burn-in applies patterns to exercise the components throughout the burn-in period.

Once the appropriate type of burn-in is determined, the location for the burn-in must be decided. Most component manufacturers can provide pre-screened and burned-in parts at a cost slightly above the cost of non-burned-in components. Device manufacturers could also perform the burn-in, if they have the proper equipment. Finally, independent test houses will burn-in components to the user's specifications. The cost and quality of all three options should be considered before a decision is made.

13.2.4 Assembly

Assembly work is done according to workmanship standards published by various industry organization or by the manufacturer. Such standards should be available in the manufacturing area for consultation where needed. No assembler should perform a task before being thoroughly familiar with the standards involved.

The assembly of a device must not reduce the reliability of the device. Special attention should be given to assure components and materials are not overstressed; lead bending, soldering and crimping are performed according to standards; burn-in must not overstress the product. Manufacturing fixtures for building or testing assemblies must be approved and validated periodically. Fixture changes must follow revision level control procedures.

Training of manufacturing personnel is also important. Training sessions should be held periodically to instruct personnel in new techniques and certify standard techniques such as soldering, crimping and static protection.

Most important, the assemblers must have a knowledge of the product they are assembling and be aware of the consequences of a bad unit. The more the assembler feels a part of the product, the better the chance they will build it reliably.

13.2.5 Test and Inspection

Subassemblies and assemblies are inspected to determine conformance to specification. Assemblies and final product are tested to assure reliable product goes out the door. All tests and inspections must be performed to agreed-upon test specifications. The specifications must assure all critical parameters are tested and any accuracy statements are confirmed. The unit is tested as thoroughly as is practically possible.

Test fixtures are built to test the unit completely, without unduly stressing it. Tests must not induce extraneous voltages, currents or pressures which would be damaging. Tests must not cause component overheating.

All test fixture documentation must be in order, including hardware and software specifications and the validation protocol. Revision level control procedures must be in effect on all fixtures. No person should operate the fixture unless they have been qualified to operate it.

13.2.6 System Burn-In

Products are collections of components which are subject to a decreasing failure rate. The manufacturing process may generate similar failure patterns, due to poor component insertion, poor soldering, bending component leads too close to the component body or the inadvertant application of electrostatic charge. Burn-in of assemblies is an effective way of improving reliability of delivered equipment. Generally, it is cheaper and more effective to burn-in the complete product, unless it is a large system made up of several testable assemblies. Sometimes, burn-in of PC boards may be performed as well, particularly for equipment where repairs at the final assembly stage would be costly. PC boards are also burned-in when used as Service replacements, because placing a non-burned-in component or assembly into a device which has been operational for some time will drastically reduce the reliability of the device. Replacement parts must always be burned-in.

Planning for system burn-in is a multi-stepped procedure, which begins with the analysis of the various components. Whether particular components are burned-in will effect any system burn-in. Failure modes and effects analysis may highlight particular components with high failure rates or those whose failure would have a serious impact on the functionality of the unit. The burn-in would then concentrate primarily on these components. Burn-in data from previous devices similar to the one under production should be reviewed. Failures should be analyzed and the procedure used as a model for the new product, with appropriate changes where necessary.

System burn-in should be an integral part of the pilot build of units. It is of the utmost importance that the times-to-failure are monitored as continuously as practically possible and that the failing components are identified along with their failure mode. These failures can then be traced back to their causes, for possible changes to the process. The burn-in procedure can be adjusted accordingly. The time-to-failure information can be used to optimize the system burn-in protocol. For example, a process failure might be the bending of component leads too near the component body. This may cause material cracking, which will introduce a latent defect. By accelerated burn-in, this defect can be captured and the process changed prior to production release.

Burn-in should be performed in an environment that is as close as possible to the worst case combination of temperature and electrical and mechanical stresses within the product specification. The time of the burn-in should depend on the status of the various components being used and previous burn-in history of similar products. Once the parameters are established, test the burn-in procedure during initial builds, modify it based on the analysis of the failures. Having established a good confidence level in the procedure, the production procedure should yield highly reliable devices.

13.2.7 Failure Analysis

Analysis of failed parts or assemblies is extremely important. It provides feedback to the assembler and vendor on how they are performing.

The purpose of failure analysis is to determine the cause of the failure and eliminate it. Thus failure analysis should be carried to the component level. By doing so, vendor or lot problems may be determined and the appropriate action taken. Where the failure is caused by a process problem, immediate changes can be made.

It is important to keep a log of failures to serve as a means of checking performance. It speeds detection when similar type problems occur. It also provides data for plotting failure curves over a period of time.

13.2.8 Statistical Process Control

Statistical Process Control (SPC) activities should be implemented as a meanss of measuring the overall quality of the manufacturing actdivity. They also serve to improve the overall attitude of the personnel involved. Techniques, such as charts plotting performance serve to challenge the individual, foster competition and improve the attitude of the individuals, resulting in a higher quality product.

13.2.9 Electrostatic Discharge Protection

Electrostatic discharge (ESD) has become a major problem in electronic manufacturing in recent years. Static electricity, created by materials and movement within manufacturing and design areas, can damage sensitive electronic components and costs manufacturers millions of dollars each year.

The trend in electronics is toward smaller, faster microelectronic components that use less power. The increase in sensitivity has left these components, in some cases, highly susceptible to static-induced damage. The metal oxide semiconductor (MOS) technology, for example, has produced devices that are particularly vulnerable. The threshold of sensitivity for such components as VMOS-type semiconductors is in the range of 30 to 40 volts.

Other static-sensitive devices include:

Junction field-effect transistors
Some bipolar devices
Diodes
Thick-film resistors.

Within such components, static electricity can cause short-circuiting, electrical breakdown of the gate oxide or changes in critical values. Degradation of components caused by static is difficult to identify and may not be discovered until premature failures occur in the field. Some manufacturers believe there are ten degraded components for each one damaged.

Antistatic control together with operator training should be implemented in all manufacturing areas. Such controls include:

Wrist and heel straps
Ionization systems
Antistatic sprays
Floor and table mats
Special clothing
Special flooring or carpets.

Operator training, use of antistatic devices and facility modifications are three measures that not only reduce component damage but also raise worker productivity.

13.3 The FDA and GMP

The FDA promulgated the Good Manufacturing Practices (GMP) for medical devices regulations in 1978, drawing authority from the Medical Device Amendments to the Federal Food, Drug and Cosmetic Act of 1976. The GMP regulations represented a total quality assurance program intended to control the manufacture and distribution of devices. It allows the FDA to periodically inspect medical device manufacturers.

The GMP specifies general objectives, e.g., calibrated equipment, process controls, control of packaging and labeling rather than methods, since one method might not be applicable to all manufacturing processes. In most cases, it is left to the manufacturer to determine the best method to attain these objectives. In some cases, the GMP does specify the particular type of method to be used. A manufacturer may, however, vary from this method, if the intent of the GMP requirement is met.

All manufacturers of medical devices must establish and implement a GMP program under the general umbrella of the medical device GMP regulation, that is specific to the nature of the device.

13.3.1 Written Procedures

The GMP requires written procedures for certain processes. The purpose of these written procedures is to provide guidance, to assure uniformity and completeness, and for communicating and managing operations. Often training and work experience are valid substitutes for written procedures. Typically, a written procedure may not be necessary when:

> The activity is very simple
>
> Straightforward quantitative rather than qualitative standards determine acceptability
>
> The operation is performed by skilled personnel

13.3.2 Application of the GMP

The medical device Good Manufacturing Practices applies to the manufacture of finished devices and equipment intended for human use. The GMP is not intended to apply to manufacturers of components, although such manufacturers are encouraged to use appropriate provisions of the regulation as guidelines. The GMP applies to the design and control of facilities, production and measurement equipment and the production process. The GMP does not, however, apply to the quantification of the device design to assure it is safe and effective. The GMP assumes the device design reflects a safe and effective device, fit for its intended purpose. Once the design is verified and qualified, the GMP's contributions to assuring a safe and effective device is in maintaining the intrinsic safety and effectiveness established during the design phase. The GMPs do, however, address design retrospectively, through such requirements as the complaint file and failure investigations.

The GMP regulations address all areas of the manufacturing processes, including:

> Organization and personnel
> Buildings
> Equipment
> Control of components
> Production and process control
> Packaging and labeling control
> Holding, distribution and installation
> Device evaluation
> Records.

13.3.3 Quality Assurance Requirements

All manufacturers of medical devices and medical equipment must establish and implement a Quality Assurance program appropriate to the product which is manufactured. Such a program consists of all the applicable requirements of the GMP, and any additional controls necessary to assure that the finished device, manufacturing process and all related procedures conform to approved specifications.

The GMP is based on Quality Assurance principles and was designed to prevent the production of nonconforming products. The GMP assures that quality controls are provided for those processes and activities that affect quality.

13.3.4 GMP Inspections

The FDA will inspect a facility at least once every two years. During the inspections, investigators look for company knowledge, control and quality audits. FDA operates a two track system of GMP inspections. The two tracks detail the depth to which an inspection is conducted.

Track I inspections are the less detailed of the two types. A Track I inspection typically examines:

> Complaint handling
> Failure investigations
> Change control procedures
> Auditing practices
> New technologies or products
> Changes in the Quality Assurance system
> Recalls.

The inspection will be Track I if all of the following conditions are met:

> A comprehensive GMP inspection was conducted in the last four years and the inspection revealed no serious problems
>
> The firm has an adequate quality history
>
> There was a satisfactory evaluation of product or process changes during the last GMP inspection
>
> If samples were collected during the last GMP inspection, and the classification of those samples did not reveal any significant quality assurance problems.

Track II inspections are similar to Track I, except the inspection is much more detailed and will generally last longer. The investigator will require more information and will spend much of the inspection time in the manufacturing area.

13.3.4.1 Details of the Inspection

The most critical part of an inspection is FDA's review of a firm's complaint handling. This review will encompass an examination of the procedures a firm has established, a selected sample of complaints and the actions taken by a firm in response to those specific complaints.

A second key point in the inspection is a firm's failure investigation and analysis system. Investigators will determine whether there is a formally documented failure analysis program adequate to:

> Develop a trend analysis
> Identify problem causes
> Determine the significance of a defect
> Initiate a design review, as needed
> Determine the impact on related products
> Establish corrective actions.

The investigator will also review failure investigation and analysis records for the past two years to determine whether the firm adequately accomplished identifying problem areas, evaluating the significance of defects and following-up on corrective actions, where appropriate.

A third key point in the inspection is a firm's change control procedures. In determining whether a firm's change control procedures are adequate, the areas to be considered include:

> Component and finished device specifications
> Manufacturing procedures and specifications
> Records.

A fourth point in the inspection is audit evaluation. The investigator will determine whether:

> The firm has written procedures
> The procedures are adequate
> The firm follows its audit schedule.

A fifth area to be evaluated is changes or additions to the product line, in manufacturing or to the quality assurance system. This review includes a plant walk-through and questioning of management.

Finally, an inspector will look for any recalls previously unknown to the FDA. If the firm had a significant recall since the last inspection that was not brought to FDA's attention, the investigator will want to see records pertaining to that recall and will interview management about the corrective action that was taken and whether the recall has been completed.

Records from most FDA GMP inspections, including information from complaint files, are available under the Freedom of Information Act to competitors and plaintiffs in a product liability suit. The firm may request certain parts of a record be kept confidential, but there is no guarantee this request will be honored. Similarly, internal compliance documents, including as quality audits and complaints, are also available to plaintiffs through discovery in a product liability action.

Failure to meet FDA's GMP regulations might constitute evidence of negligence and could be used against a company. Moreover, internal memoranda relating to GMP inspections often contain damaging statements concerning the adequacy of a company's GMP program and, by implication, the safety and effectiveness of its products. Companies should establish a Record Retention Policy which details the periodic review and purging of files to remove non-required, potentially damaging documents.

When the results of the inspection include adverse findings, the inspector lists them on FDA Form 483 and discusses them during the exit interview. The 483 becomes part of the FDA's file on the firm. The company has the right to formally respond to the 483.

13.3.5 Sanctions

The FDA may impose sanctions for non-compliance with GMP regulations, including:

> More frequent inspections
> Issuance of Regulatory Letters
> Notices of adverse findings
> Product recalls
> Product seizures and detentions
> Operation injunctions
> Criminal prosecution.

13.4 Summary

Manufacturers must operate in an environment in which the manufacturing process is controlled. Manufacturing excellence can only be achieved by designing products and processes to address potential problems before they occur. Manufacturers must also operate in an enviroment that meets GMP regulations established by the FDA. This requires proof of control over manufacturing processes and field information.

Once the device is manufactured, field information becomes an important source of product information, which is invaluable to the designer and to Reliability Assurance. Methods of obtaining and structuring such information is discussed in the next chapter.

13.5 References

1. Boxleitner, W., "Removing 'Black Magic' From Your ESD Tests," *Test and Measurement World*. September, 1987.

2. Burgess, J. A., *Design Assurance for Engineers and Managers*. New York: Marcel Dekker, 1984.

3. CDRH, *Medical Device GMP Guidance for FDA Investigators*. Washington, DC: U.S. Department of Health and Human Services, 1984.

4. Connors, T. J., "The Cost of Screening vs Not Screening," *Evaluation Engineering*. July-August, 1987.

5. Dash, G. and I. Straus, "ESD Testing and Design at the System Level," *Compliance Engineering*. 1989 Reference Guide.

6. Dash, G. and I. Straus, "Static Control in the Manufacturing Process," *Compliance Engineering*. 1989 Reference Guide.

7. Duncan, A. J., *Quality Control and Industrial Statistics*. Homewood, Illinois: Richard D. Irwin, Inc., 1974.

8. Heidenreich, P., "Designing for Manufacturability," *Quality Progress*. May, 1988.

9. Jacobs, D. M., "ESD: A Primer," *Quality Progress*. March, 1988.

10. Jensen, F. and N. E. Peterson, *Burn-In*. New York: John Wiley and Sons, 1982.

11. Johnson, L. M., *Quality Assurance Program Evaluation*. Stockton Trade Press, Inc., 1982.

12. MIL-STD-105, *Sampling Procedures and Tables for Inspection by Attributes*. Washington, DC: Department of Defense, 1963.

13. Pratt, D. and J. Davis, "Can Your Product Survive Real-World ESD?," *Test and Measurement World*. December, 1988.

14. Ross, R., "Solving Static Electricity Problems In the Manufacturing Environment," *Electronic Manufacturing*. April, 1989.

14

The Field Operation Phase

The goal of the Product Development process is to put a safe, effective and reliable medical device in the hands of a physician or other medical personnel where it may be used to improve health care. The company has designed and manufactured the device to be safe, effective and reliable. They have warrantied the device for a certain period of time, usually one year. Is this the end of the firm's concern for the device? It shouldn't be. There is too much valuable information to be obtained.

When a product is subjected to a reliability program during design and development, testing is performed to determine the degree of reliability present in the device and the confidence in that determination. There is, however, no guarantee that the product, as manufactured and shipped, has that same degree of reliability. The most meaningful way to determine the degree of reliablity within each device is to monitor its activity in the field.

Analysis of field data is the only means of determining how a product is performing in actual use. It is a means of determining reliability growth over time. It is a measure of how well the product was specified, designed and manufactured. It is a source of information on the effectiveness of the shipping configuration. It is also a source of data for product enhancements or new designs.

Field information may be obtained in any of several ways, including:

Analysis of Field Service Reports
Failure Analysis of Failed Units
Warranty Analysis.

14.1 Analysis of Field Service Reports

The type of data necessary for a meaningful analysis of product reliability is gathered from Field Service Reports. These reports contain valuable information, such as:

Type of product
Serial number
Date of service activity
Symptom of the problem
Diagnosis
List of parts replaced
Labor hours required
Service representative.

The type of product allows classification of reports by individual model. The serial number allows a history of each individual unit to be established and provides traceability to the manufacturing date. The date of service activity helps to indicate the length of time since the last Service activity or since the manufacturing date.

The symptom is the problem, as recognized by the user. The diagnosis is the description of the cause of the problem from analysis by the service representative. It should be noted that the cause of the problem may be remote from the user's original complaint. The list of parts replaced is an adjunct to the diagnosis and can serve to trend parts usage and possible vendor problems.

The required labor hours help in evaluating the complexity of a problem, as represented by the time involved in repair. It, along with the name of the Service Representative, acts as a check on the efficiency of the individual representative, as average labor hours for the same failure code may be compared on a representative to representative basis. The labor hours per problem may be calculated to assist in determining warranty cost as well as determining the efficiency of service methods.

Additional data necessary for analysis is the date of manufacture of each unit and the length of time between manufacture and the time that the problem occurred. The manufacturing date is kept on file in the Device History Record. The length of time since manufacture is calculated by subtracting the manufacturing date from the date of service.

14.1.1 The Database

Field Service Reports are sorted by product upon receipt. The report is scanned for completeness. Service representatives may be contacted if clarification of an entry or lack of information would lead to an incomplete database record. The diagnoses are coded, according to a list of failures, as developed by Reliability Assurance, Design Engineering and

Manufacturing Engineering (Figure 14.1). Manufacturing date and the length of time since manufacture are obtained.

Figure 14.1 List of Failure Codes

Base Machine

101	Missing Parts
102	Shipping Damage
103	Circuit Breaker Wiring Defect
104	Regulator Defect
105	Shelf Latch Broken

Monitor

201	Display Problems
202	Control Cable Defect
203	Power Board Problem
204	Control Board Problem
205	Unstable Reference Voltage

The data is entered into a computer data base, where it may be manipulated to determine the necessary parameters. Each Field Service Report is input to a single database record, unless the service report contains multiple failure codes. Figure 15.2 shows a sample database record.

The data is first sorted by service date, so trending can be accomplished by a predetermined time period, such as a fiscal quarter. Data within that time frame is then sorted by problem code, indicating the frequency of problems during the particular reporting period. A pareto analysis of the problems can then be developed. Data is finally sorted by serial number, which gives an indication of which devices experienced multiple service call and or experienced continuing problems.

Percentages of each problem type as part of the total number of problems reported are helpful in determining primary failures. Spread sheets are developed listing the problems versus manufacturing dates (Figure 14.3) and the problems versus time since manufacturing (Figure 14.4). The spread sheet data can then be plotted and analyzed.

14.1.2 Data Analysis

The most important reason for collecting the field data is to extract significant problem information and structure it so that the cause of prod-

Figure 14.2 Sample Database Record

Field	Field Name	Type of Field	Width
1	SERVICEDATE	Numeric	4
2	SERIALNUM	Character	9
3	MANUFDATE	Numeric	4
4	USETIME	Character	3
5	FAILCODE	Character	4
6	PARTS1	Character	13
7	PARTS2	Character	13
8	PARTS3	Character	13
9	PARTS4	Character	13
10	PARTS5	Character	13
11	LABORHRS	Numeric	4
12	REPNO	Numeric	4

Figure 14.3 Problems versus Manufacturing Date

Manufacture Date	Failure Code						Total
	153	154	202	225	305	401	
1/88	0	0	0	0	0	0	0
2/88	8	2	0	0	1	1	12
3/88	13	0	0	2	4	7	26
4/88	3	0	3	0	4	0	10
5/88	1	1	0	7	1	2	12
6/88	9	3	2	4	2	3	23
7/88	0	3	1	0	2	2	7
8/88	6	5	3	4	3	1	22
9/88	5	8	12	4	3	4	36
10/88	0	3	2	2	7	0	14
11/88	3	5	6	3	2	3	22
12/88	5	7	9	8	8	12	49

Figure 14.4 Problems versus Time Since Manufacture

Number of Months	Failure Code						Total
	153	154	202	225	305	401	
1	1	3	2	0	2	0	8
2	2	3	8	5	6	4	27
3	2	3	2	5	1	1	14
4	1	1	3	0	0	2	7
5	0	2	1	1	2	1	7
6	1	1	4	2	0	3	11
7	1	2	3	4	2	2	14
8	2	2	3	8	4	4	23
9	3	2	4	18	3	9	39
10	2	3	4	12	3	6	30
11	1	3	2	2	0	3	11
12	1	1	2	2	0	0	6

uct problems may be highlighted, trended, analyzed and corrected. The cause of the problem must be determined and the most appropriate solution implemented. A "band-aid" solution is unacceptable.

Figure 14.5 Pareto Plot of Problems

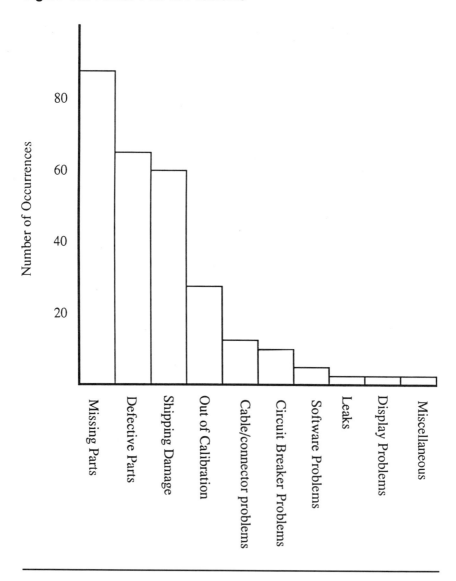

Pareto analysis is used to identify major problems. The individual problems are plotted along the x-axis and the frequency on the y-axis. The result is a histogram of problems, where the severity of the problem is indicated, leading to the establishment of priorities in addressing solutions (Figure 14.5).

Several graphical plots are helpful in analyzing problems. One is the plot of particular problems versus length of time since manufacturing. This plot is used to determine the area of the life cycle in which the problem occurs. Peaks of problem activity indicate infant mortality, useful life or wearout, depending on the length of time since manufacture (Figure 14.6).

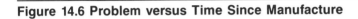

Figure 14.6 Problem versus Time Since Manufacture

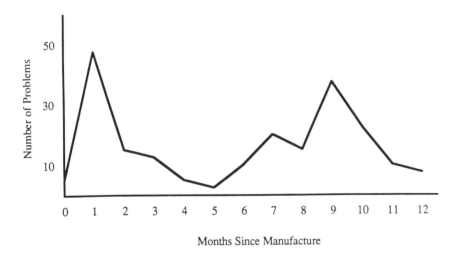

A second plot of interest is that of a particular problem versus the date of manufacture (Figure 14.7). This plot is a good indication of the efficiency of the manufacturing process. It shows times where problems occur, e.g., the rush to ship product at the end of a fiscal quarter, lot problems on components or vendor problems The extent of the problem is an indication of the correct or incorrect solution.

Another useful plot is that of the total number of problems versus the date of manufacture (Figure 14.8). The learning curve for the product is visible at the peaks of the curve. It can also be shown how the

Figure 14.7 Problem versus Date of Manufacture

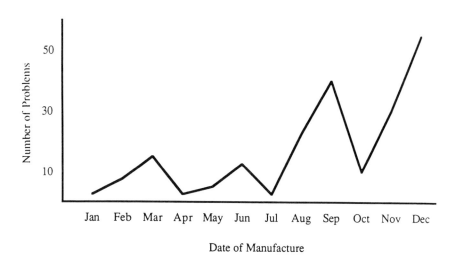

Figure 14.8 Problems versus Date of Manufacture

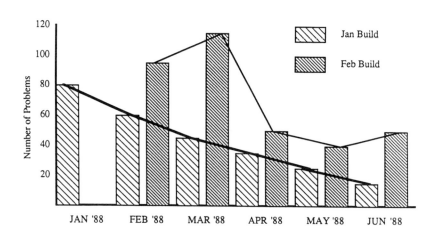

problems for subsequent builds decrease as manufacturing personnel become more familiar and efficient with the process.

Trending of problems, set against the time of reporting (Figure 14.9) is an indicator of the extent of a problem and the effectiveness of corrective action. Decreasing numbers indicate the solution is effective. Reappearing high counts indicate the initial solution did not address the cause of the problem.

Figure 14.9 Problem Trending

Problem	1/89	2/89	3/89	4/89	5/89	6/89	7/89	8/89	9/89	Total	% Total
Case Cracked	0	0	0	1	2	2	0	0	0	5	5.2
Broken Hinge	0	0	0	0	0	1	3	0	0	4	4.2
Bent Pin	0	0	1	1	0	0	0	2	2	6	6.3
Broken Wire	2	7	0	2	1	2	0	0	0	14	14.7
Leak	1	2	1	0	0	0	1	2	0	7	7.4
Bad O-Ring	3	4	1	1	3	2	5	3	4	26	27.4
U2 Bad	0	0	1	1	2	2	0	0	0	6	6.3
Bad Switch	0	0	0	3	4	4	2	3	1	17	17.9
Bad Jack	0	0	0	1	3	2	3	1	0	10	10.5
Total	6	13	4	10	15	15	14	11	7	95	

The database is also useful for analyzing warranty costs. The data can be used to calculate warranty expenses, problems per manufactured unit and warranty costs as a percentage of sales (Figure 14.10).

A similar table can be established for installation of devices.

14.2 Failure Analysis of Field Units

Most failure analysis performed in the field is done at the board level. Service Representative usually solve problems by board swapping, since they are not equipped to troubleshoot at the component level. Boards should be returned from the field to be analyzed to the component level.

Figure 14.10 Warranty Analysis — Evaluation of Costs

Product Code	Parameters	January 1988	February 1988	Year to Date
4423	Normal Warranty	$9458.00	$3017.00	$12475.00
	Recall Warranty	$630.00	$0.00	$630.00
	Total Warranty	$10088.00	$3017.00	$13105.00
	Setup Cost	$7522.00	$3130.00	$10652.00
	Total Cost	$17610.00	$6147.00	$23757.00
	Sales	$189228.00	$312677.00	$501905.00
	Warranty/Sales	5.0%	1.0%	2.5%
	Setup/Sales	4.0%	1.0%	2.1%
	Total/Sales	9.3%	2.0%	4.7%
	# Units Shipped	38	62	100
	# Units Setup	25	17	42
	# Warranty Units	32	17	49
	# Recall Units	2	0	2
	Warranty/Unit	$295.56	$177.47	$254.59
	Recall/Unit	$315.00	$0.00	$315.00
	Setup/Unit	$300.88	$184.12	$253.62
	Total/Unit	$298.47	$180.79	$255.45

This not only yields data for trending purposes, but highlights the real cause of the problem. It also gives data on problem parts or problem vendors.

The most important process in performing field failure analysis is focusing on the cause of the problem, based on the symptom. It does little good to develop a fix for a symptom if the cause is not known. To do so only creates additional problems. Analysis techniques, such as fault tree analysis or Failure Modes and Effects Analysis may help to focus on the cause.

Once the component level analysis is completed, pareto charts may be made, highlighting problem areas and prioritizing solutions. The major problems can be placed in a spread sheet, similar to that shown in

Figure 14.9, and monitored over time. Graphical plots, similar to that
shown in Figure 14.6, can also be drawn to monitor various parameters
over time.

14.3 Warranty Analysis

Warranty analysis is an indication of the reliability of a device in its
early life, usually the first year. Warranty analysis (Figure 14.10) is a
valuable source of information on such parameters as warranty cost as
a percentage of sales, warranty cost per unit, installation cost per unit
and percentage of shipped units experiencing problems. By plotting this
data, a trend can be established over time.

14.4 The GMP and Field Data

GMP regulations contain requirements for several activities involved
with field data, including:

> Complaint handling
> Medical Device Reporting
> Failure investigation
> Trending
> Product recalls.

14.4.1 Complaint Handling

A procedure must be in place which distinguishes between routine service and complaints. Typically, requests for service and repair need not
be considered as complaints when they are routine requests for maintenance, adjustment or repair of damage or failure resulting from long
use, misuse or accident.

All repair or service requests that result from failure of a device to
perform its intended function due to design defects or to inadequate design, unanticipated component failure or other causes of a non-routine
nature must be evaluated as candidates for the complaint file.

In examining a firm's complaint handling procedures, the FDA will
want to know whether the complaint handling system:

> Provides guidance as to the definition of a complaint

> Assigns responsibility for handling complaints

> Provides instructions for obtaining and documenting com-
> plaint information

> Provides instructions for investigational follow-up

Provides methods for collecting, analyzing and evaluating data

Provides criteria for determining events that are reportable under the Medical Device Reporting (MDR) regulation

Includes files that are maintained properly

Provides exhibits of required forms.

The inspector will also want to determine that:

The complaint file was adequately reviewed, evaluated and, if necessary, investigated

The records contain the reason(s) why and the name of the responsible individual, if the decision was made not to investigate

The complaint was immediately reviewed, evaluated and investigated by a designated individual if the complaint pertained to an injury, death or any hazard to safety.

Investigations are carried out to the degree necessary to draw conclusions as to the validity and cause of the complaint. A review of the Device History Record should be made, as appropriate.

Where an investigation was made, the record of investigation includes:

Name of the device
Any control numbers utilized
Name of the complainant
Nature of the complaint
Result of the firm's investigation
Recommended corrective action, if any
Reply to the complainant.

14.4.2 Medical Device Reporting (MDR)

Medical Device Reporting requires that a manufacturer or importer report to the FDA whenever it "receives or otherwise becomes aware of information that reasonably suggests that one of its marketed devices 1) may have caused or contributed to a death or serious injury or 2) has malfunctioned and that the device or any other device marketed by the manufacturer or importer would be likely to cause or contribute to a death or serious injury if the malfunction were to recur."

A serious injury is defined as an injury "that is 1) life threatening,

2) results in permanent impairment of a body function or permanent damage to body structure or 3) necessitates medical or surgical intervention by a health care professional."

The Medical Device Reporting regulation requires reports to be filed within specified time periods from learning about an event. In many cases this occurs before the firm has time to investigate the situation. Death or serious injury reports must be filed within five calendar days and malfunction reports within fifteen working days of learning about the event. Reports must be filed even if the event arose from deliberate or inadvertant misuse.

It is difficult to generalize with respect to what is and what is not reportable with respect to events in foreign countries. Each situation merits careful attention and a decision reached based only on a careful analysis of the regulation as applied to the specific facts. As a general rule, if a U.S. company learns that one of its devices manufactured in the U.S. but sold abroad has caused a reportable event, it must report that event. If a U.S. firm has a subsidiary that manufacturesd a product abroad and that product has only been sold abroad, an event associated with that device is not required to be reported to the FDA.

Medical Device Reporting information is available to competitors or plaintiff's attorneys through Freedom of Information (FOI).

14.4.3 Failure Investigation

A firm must have a formally documented failure analysis program adequate to identify problem causes, determine the significance of a defect, determine the impact on related products and establish corrective actions. An investigator will always determine whether the corrective was completed.

14.4.4 Trending

Trending of field data, such as complaints or field failures, provides information on the extent of the problem and on the success of the solution. It also meets GMP regulations.

14.4.5 Product Recalls

A recall is "a firm's removal or correction of a marketed product that the FDA considers to be in violation of the laws it administers and against which the agency would initiate legal action." Recalls are classified relative to the degree of health hazard presented by the product being recalled:

Class I   A situation in which there is a reasonable probability
                 that the use of or exposure to a violative product will
                 cause serious adverse health consequences or death

Class II   A situation in which the use of or exposure to a viola-
                 tive product may cause temporary or medically reversi-
                 ble adverse health consequences or where the probabil-
                 ity of serious adverse health consequences is remote

Class III   A situation in which the use of or exposure to a viola-
                 tive product is not likely to cause adverse health conse-
                 quences

Recalls are voluntary actions initiated by the recalling firm. As a general rule, the FDA lacks the legal authority to mandate that a firm recall a violative product, although it may pressure the firm into a 'voluntary' recall.

FDA guidelines set forth a number of actions or procedures a firm
is requested to follow, including:

> Health hazard evaluation
> Development of a recall strategy
> Preparation of status reports

The status reports will be monitored by the FDA and they will notify
the firm when they feel the recall is complete.

14.5 Summary

Analysis of field data is the means of determining how well a device
is performing in its actual environment. Analysis also provides information on failures, the manufacturing learning curve, manufacturing
process problems, trends of failures and warranty costs. FDA regulations
also require complaint investigations, failure investigations, trending
and Medical Device Reporting.

This information is of little value unless it is made available to appropriate departments within the company that need it. Feedback is the
last phase in the development cycle.

14.6 References

1. AAMI, *Guideline for Establishing and Administering Medical In-
     strumentation*. Arlington, Virginia: Association for the Advance-
     ment of Medical Instrumentation, 1984.

2. Fries, R. C. et. al., "A Reliability Assurance Database for Analysis of Medical Product Performance," *Proceedings of the Symposium on the Engineering of Computer-Based Medical Systems.* New York: The Institute of Electrical and Electronic Engineers, 1988.

3. MIL-HDBK-472, *Maintainability Prediction.* Washington, DC: Department of Defense, 1966.

4. 21 CFR 7

5. 21 CFR 803

6. 21 CFR 807

7. 21 CFR 812

15

The Feedback Phase

The feedback phase is the final phase in the development process. It is the phase that forms the link between the designers and the field. Referring again to the product life cycle (Figure 15.1), feedback relates the field data to the appropriate personnel for analysis and possible future action.

Figure 15.1 Product Life Cycle

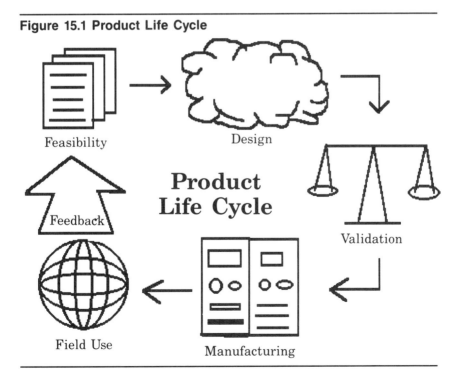

Feasibility

Design

Product Life Cycle

Feedback

Validation

Field Use

Manufacturing

Several areas require this feedback:

Engineering
Manufacturing Engineering
Regulatory Affairs
Reliability Assurance
Quality Assurance
Marketing
Legal
Top Management.

15.1 Engineering

Engineering needs to know what problems in the field are caused by improper design, unanticipated usage or insufficient safety margin. Engineering personnel also assist other groups with their problems, as the engineers know the design better than anyone. Engineering will take the data and decide if design changes are needed or whether future enhancements will decrease warranty costs or increase sales.

15.2 Manufacturing Engineering

Manufacturing Engineering needs to know what problems are caused by insufficient manufacturing processes or incomplete manufacturing tests. They will take the data and decide if changes to the manufacturing procedures or additional tests are necessary.

15.3 Regulatory Affairs

Under the GMP's, product complaints must be kept on file as well as Medical Device Reporting (MDR) for failures involving injury or death to a patient or user. For this reason, Regulatory Affairs must be aware of field problems and establish a system to determine if the problems are complaints or are candidates for a MDR.

15.4 Reliability Assurance

Reliability Assurance has established a MTBF value during its preshipment testing. By analyzing data from the field, the growth of that MTBF value can be tracked. The GMPs require trending of field data to detect problem trends. This usually falls into the realm of Reliability Assurance.

15.5 Quality Assurance

Field data will indicate to Quality Assurance whether problems are caused by a bad lot of components, vendor problems, deviations from specification, insufficient burn-in or inadequate shipping containers. Quality Assurance will review the information and take appropriate action to correct the problems.

15.6 Marketing

Marketing needs to know how the device is meeting the customer's expectations and what, if any, problems are occurring. By looking at summary reports of the field data, they can be aware of what is happening in the field and hold more meaningful discussion with physicians and other medical personnel.

15.7 Legal

With the use of a medical device, there is always the possibility of legal action being taken for a problem caused by the device. The Legal department must be aware of what problems are occurring and by working with Regulatory Affairs and Reliability Assurance, determine what problems might lead to legal action and the seriousness of the situation.

15.8 Top Management

The success of a business depend on the success of each of its products. There is a maxim in reliability that states the reliability of a product is proportional to its least reliable component. I would suggest that the reliability of a company is dependent on its least reliable product. When a product is considered unreliable by its users, the company reputation suffers, no matter how good the rest of its products are. Therefore, top management needs to be aware of how the device is being accepted in the field, what problems there are and how the device is affecting the bottom line. This data will be needed for future decisions on the life of a product, enhancements and new product introductions.

15.9 Summary

Feedback completes the product life cycle in that data from the field causes the life cycle to begin anew. Whether the data indicates changes or enhancements to devices or processes, the feasibility of the activity must be analyzed, the activity must be designed, validated, implemented and then monitored. Feedback may then cause further change or enhancement.

Medical device development is an evolutionary process, constantly working towards improving the health care of all individuals. Reliability is a philosophy which structures the way the process is approached. Reliability not only involves making the device safe and effective, it more importantly involves making the process and the people working within that process safe and effective. If the process and the people are reliable, the device will be too.

The philosophy of reliability has been stated best by Dr. Dimitri Kececioglu at the University of Arizona in his classes and seminars. He states that everyone needs to develop PRIDE in all their activities. PRIDE stands for Putting Reliability Into Daily Efforts. If everyone adopted this philosophy, the benefits would be enormous.

Appendix 1

Chi-Square Table

Figure Appendix 1

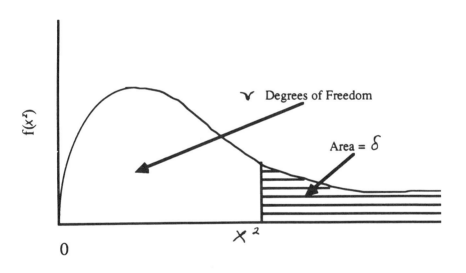

ν/∂	0.975	0.950	0.900	0.050	0.100	0.050	0.025
1	0.001	0.004	0.016	0.455	2.706	3.841	5.024
2	0.051	0.103	0.211	1.386	4.605	5.991	7.378
3	0.216	0.352	0.584	2.366	6.251	7.815	9.348
4	0.484	0.711	1.064	3.357	7.779	9.488	11.143
5	0.831	1.145	1.610	4.351	9.236	11.070	12.832
6	1.237	1.635	2.204	5.348	10.645	12.592	14.449
7	1.690	2.167	2.833	6.346	12.017	14.067	16.013
8	2.180	2.733	3.490	7.344	13.362	15.507	17.535
9	2.700	3.325	4.168	8.343	14.684	16.919	19.023
10	3.247	3.940	4.865	9.342	15.987	18.307	20.483
11	3.816	4.575	5.578	10.341	17.275	19.675	21.920
12	4.404	5.226	6.304	11.340	18.549	21.026	23.337
13	5.009	5.892	7.042	12.340	19.812	22.362	24.736
14	5.629	6.571	7.790	13.339	21.064	23.685	26.119
15	6.262	7.261	8.547	14.339	22.307	24.996	27.488
16	6.908	7.962	9.312	15.338	23.542	26.296	28.845
17	7.564	8.672	10.085	16.338	24.769	27.587	30.191
18	8.231	9.390	10.865	17.338	25.989	28.869	31.526
19	8.907	10.117	11.651	18.338	27.204	30.144	32.852
20	9.591	10.851	12.443	19.337	28.412	31.410	34.170
21	10.283	11.591	13.240	20.337	29.615	32.671	35.479
22	10.982	12.338	14.041	21.337	30.813	33.924	36.781
23	11.688	13.091	14.848	22.337	32.007	35.172	38.076
24	12.401	13.848	15.659	23.337	33.196	36.415	39.364
25	13.120	14.611	16.473	24.337	34.382	37.652	40.646
26	13.844	15.379	17.292	25.336	35.563	38.885	41.923
27	14.573	16.151	18.114	26.336	36.741	40.113	43.194
28	15.308	16.928	18.939	27.336	37.916	41.337	44.461
29	16.047	17.708	19.768	28.336	39.087	42.557	45.722
30	16.791	18.493	20.599	29.336	40.256	43.773	46.979

Appendix 2

Percent Rank Tables

The table lists the percentile points of order statistics in random samples from a uniform distribution. The median rank (50.0) is the value the true probability of failure should have with 50% confidence at the time of the kth failure in N units. The 10%/90%, 5%/95% and 2.5%/97.5% ranks are used to plot the lower and upper confidence limits on the cumulative distribution function.

Sample Size = 1

Order Number	2.5	5.0	10.0	50.0	90.0	95.0	97.5
1	2.500	5.000	10.000	50.000	90.000	95.000	97.500

Sample Size = 2

Order Number	2.5	5.0	10.0	50.0	90.0	95.0	97.5
1	1.258	2.532	5.132	29.289	68.377	77.639	84.189
2	15.811	22.361	31.623	71.711	94.868	97.468	98.742

Sample Size = 3

Order Number	2.5	5.0	10.0	50.0	90.0	95.0	97.5
1	0.840	1.695	3.451	20.630	53.584	63.160	70.760
2	9.430	13.535	19.580	50.000	80.420	86.465	90.570
3	29.240	36.840	46.416	79.370	96.549	98.305	99.160

Sample Size = 4

Order Number	2.5	5.0	10.0	50.0	90.0	95.0	97.5
1	0.631	1.274	2.600	15.910	43.766	52.713	60.236
2	6.759	9.761	14.256	38.573	67.954	75.140	80.588
3	19.412	24.860	32.046	61.427	85.744	90.239	93.241
4	39.764	47.287	56.234	84.090	97.400	98.726	99.369

Sample Size = 5

Order Number	2.5	5.0	10.0	50.0	90.0	95.0	97.5
1	0.505	1.021	2.085	12.945	36.904	45.072	52.182
2	5.274	7.644	11.223	31.381	58.389	65.741	71.642
3	14.663	18.926	24.664	50.000	75.336	81.074	85.337
4	28.358	34.259	41.611	68.619	88.777	92.356	94.726
5	47.818	54.928	63.096	87.055	97.915	98.979	99.495

Sample Size = 6

Order Number	2.5	5.0	10.0	50.0	90.0	95.0	97.5
1	0.421	0.851	1.741	19.910	31.871	39.304	45.926
2	4.327	6.285	9.260	26.445	51.032	58.180	64.123
3	11.812	15.316	20.091	42.141	66.681	72.866	77.722
4	22.278	27.134	33.319	57.859	79.909	84.684	88.188
5	35.877	41.820	48.968	73.555	90.740	93.715	95.673
6	54.074	60.696	68.129	89.090	98.259	99.149	99.579

Sample Size = 7

Order Number	2.5	5.0	10.0	50.0	90.0	95.0	97.5
1	0.361	0.730	1.494	9.428	28.031	34.816	40.962
2	3.669	5.338	7.882	22.849	45.256	52.070	57.872
3	9.899	12.876	16.964	36.412	59.618	65.874	70.958
4	18.405	22.532	27.860	50.000	72.140	77.468	81.595
5	29.042	34.126	40.382	63.588	83.036	87.124	90.101
6	42.128	47.930	54.744	77.151	92.118	94.662	96.331
7	59.038	65.184	71.969	90.752	98.506	99.270	99.639

Sample Size = 8

Order Number	2.5	5.0	10.0	50.0	90.0	95.0	97.5
1	0.316	0.639	1.308	8.300	25.011	31.234	36.942
2	3.185	4.639	6.863	20.113	40.625	47.068	52.651
3	8.523	11.111	14.685	32.052	53.822	59.969	65.086
4	15.701	19.290	23.966	44.016	65.538	71.076	75.514
5	24.486	28.924	43.462	55.984	76.034	80.710	84.299
6	34.914	40.031	46.178	67.948	85.315	88.889	91.477
7	47.349	52.932	59.375	79.887	93.137	95.361	96.815
8	63.058	68.766	74.989	91.700	98.692	99.361	99.684

Sample Size = 9

Order Number	2.5	5.0	10.0	50.0	90.0	95.0	97.5
1	0.281	0.568	1.164	7.413	22.574	28.313	33.627
2	2.814	4.102	6.077	17.962	36.836	42.914	48.250
3	7.485	9.775	12.950	28.624	49.008	54.964	60.009
4	13.700	16.875	21.040	39.308	59.942	65.506	70.070
5	21.201	25.137	30.097	50.000	69.903	74.863	78.799
6	29.930	34.494	40.058	60.692	78.960	83.125	86.300
7	39.991	45.036	50.992	71.376	87.050	90.225	92.515
8	51.750	57.086	63.164	82.038	93.923	95.898	97.186
9	66.373	71.687	77.426	92.587	98.836	99.432	99.719

Sample Size = 10

Order Number	2.5	5.0	10.0	50.0	90.0	95.0	97.5
1	0.253	0.512	1.048	6.697	20.567	25.887	30.850
2	2.521	3.677	5.453	16.226	33.685	39.416	44.502
3	6.674	8.726	11.583	25.857	44.960	50.690	55.610
4	12.155	15.003	18.756	35.510	55.173	60.662	65.245
5	18.709	22.244	26.732	45.169	64.578	69.646	73.762
6	26.238	30.354	35.422	54.831	73.268	77.756	81.291
7	34.755	39.338	44.827	64.490	81.244	84.997	87.845
8	44.390	49.310	55.040	74.143	88.417	91.274	93.326
9	55.498	60.584	66.315	83.774	94.547	96.323	97.479
10	69.150	74.113	79.433	93.303	98.952	99.488	99.747

Sample Size = 11

Order Number	2.5	5.0	10.0	50.0	90.0	95.0	97.5
1	0.230	0.465	0.953	6.107	18.887	23.840	28.491
2	2.283	3.332	4.945	14.796	31.024	36.436	41.278
3	6.022	7.882	10.477	23.579	41.516	47.009	41.776
4	10.926	13.508	16.923	32.380	51.076	56.437	60.974
5	16.749	19.958	24.053	41.189	59.947	65.019	69.210
6	23.379	27.125	31.772	50.000	68.228	72.875	76.621
7	30.790	34.981	40.053	58.811	75.947	80.042	83.251
8	39.026	43.563	48.924	67.620	83.077	86.492	89.074
9	48.224	52.991	58.484	76.421	89.523	92.118	93.978
10	58.722	63.564	68.976	85.204	95.055	96.668	97.717
11	71.509	76.160	81.113	93.893	99.047	99.535	99.770

Sample Size = 12

Order Number	2.5	5.0	10.0	50.0	90.0	95.0	97.5
1	0.211	0.427	0.874	5.613	17.460	22.092	26.465
2	2.086	3.046	4.524	13.598	28.750	33.868	38.480
3	5.486	7,187	9.565	21.669	38.552	43.811	48.414
4	9.925	12.285	15.419	29.758	47.527	52.733	57.186
5	15.165	18.102	21.868	37.853	55.900	60.914	65.112
6	21.094	24.530	28.817	45.951	63.772	68.476	72.333
7	27.667	31.524	36.228	54.049	71.183	75.470	78.906
8	34.888	39.086	44.100	62.147	78.132	81.898	84.835
9	42.814	47.267	52.473	70.242	84.581	87.715	90.075
10	51.586	56.189	61.448	78.331	90.435	92.813	94.514
11	61.520	66.132	71.250	86.402	95.476	96.954	97.914
12	73.535	77.908	82.540	94.387	99.126	99.573	99.789

Sample Size = 13

Order Number	2.5	5.0	10.0	50.0	90.0	95.0	97.5
1	0.195	0.394	0.807	5.192	16.232	20.582	24.705
2	1.921	2.805	4.169	12.579	26.784	31.634	36.030
3	5.038	6.605	8.800	20.045	35.978	41.010	45.447
4	9.092	11.267	14.161	27.528	44.426	49.465	53.813
5	13.858	16.566	20.050	35.016	52.343	57.262	61.426
6	19.223	22.396	26.373	52.508	59.824	64.520	68.422
7	25.135	28.705	33.086	50.000	66.914	71.295	74.865
8	31.578	35.480	40.176	57.492	73.627	77.604	80.777
9	38.574	42.738	47.657	64.984	79.950	83.434	86.142
10	46.187	50.535	55.574	72.472	85.839	88.733	90.908
11	54.553	58.990	64.022	79.955	91.200	93.395	94.962
12	63.970	68.366	73.216	87.421	95.831	97.195	98.079
13	75.295	79.418	83.768	94.808	99.193	99.606	99.805

Sample Size = 14

Order Number	2.5	5.0	10.0	50.0	90.0	95.0	97.5
1	0.181	0.366	0.750	4.830	15.166	19.264	23.164
2	1.779	2.600	3.866	11.702	25.067	29.673	33.868
3	4.658	6.110	8.148	18.647	33.721	38.539	42.813
4	8.389	10.405	13.094	25.608	41.698	46.566	50.798
5	12.760	15.272	18.513	32.575	49.197	54.001	58.104
6	17.661	20.607	24.316	39.544	56.311	60.959	64.862
7	23.036	26.358	30.455	46.515	63.087	67.497	71.139
8	28.861	32.503	36.913	53.485	69.545	73.642	76.964
9	35.138	39.041	43.689	60.456	75.684	79.393	82.339
10	41.896	45.999	50.803	67.425	81.487	84.728	87.240
11	49.202	53.434	58.302	74.392	86.906	89.595	91.611
12	57.187	61.461	66.279	81.353	91.852	93.890	95.342
13	66.132	70.327	74.933	88.298	96.134	97.400	98.221
14	76.836	80.736	84.834	95.170	99.250	99.634	99.819

Sample Size = 15

Order Number	2.5	5.0	10.0	50.0	90.0	95.0	97.5
1	0.169	0.341	0.700	4.516	14.230	18.104	21.802
2	1.658	2.423	3.604	10.940	23.557	27.940	31.948
3	4.331	5.685	7.586	17.432	31.279	36.344	40.460
4	7.787	9.666	12.177	23.939	39.279	43.978	48.089
5	11.824	14.166	17.197	30.452	46.397	51.075	55.100
6	16.336	19.086	22.559	36.967	53.171	57.744	61.620
7	21.267	24.373	28.218	43.483	59.647	64.043	67.713
8	26.586	29.999	34.152	50.000	65.848	70.001	73.414
9	32.287	35.957	40.353	56.517	71.782	75.627	78.733
10	38.380	42.256	46.829	63.033	77.441	80.914	83.664
11	44.900	48.925	53.603	69.548	82.803	85.834	88.176
12	51.911	56.022	60.721	76.061	87.823	90.334	92.213
13	59.540	63.656	68.271	82.568	92.414	94.315	95.669
14	68.052	72.060	76.443	89.060	96.396	97.577	98.342
15	78.198	81.896	85.770	95.484	99.300	99.659	99.831

Sample Size = 16

Order Number	2.5	5.0	10.0	50.0	90.0	95.0	97.5
1	0.158	0.320	0.656	4.240	13.404	17.075	20.591
2	1.551	2.268	3.375	10.270	22.217	26.396	30.232
3	4.047	5.315	7.097	16.365	29.956	34.383	38.348
4	7.266	9.025	11.380	22.474	37.122	41.657	45.646
5	11.017	13.211	16.056	28.589	43.892	48.440	52.377
6	15.198	17.777	21.041	34.705	50.351	54.835	58.662
7	19.753	22.669	26.292	40.823	56.544	60.899	64.565
8	24.651	27.860	31.783	46.941	62.496	66.663	70.122
9	29.878	33.337	37.504	53.059	68.217	72.140	75.349
10	35.435	39.101	43.456	59.177	73.708	77.331	80.247
11	41.338	45.165	49.649	65.295	78.959	82.223	84.802
12	47.623	51.560	56.108	71.411	83.944	86.789	88.983
13	54.354	58.343	62.878	77.526	88.620	90.975	92.734
14	61.652	65.617	70.044	83.635	92.903	94.685	95.953
15	69.768	73.604	77.783	89.730	96.625	97.732	98.449
16	79.409	82.925	86.596	95.760	99.344	99.680	99.842

Sample Size = 17

Order Number	2.5	5.0	10.0	50.0	90.0	95.0	97.5
1	0.149	0.301	0.618	3.995	12.667	16.157	19.506
2	1.458	2.132	3.173	9.678	21.021	25.012	28.689
3	3.799	4.990	6.667	15.422	28.370	32.619	36.441
4	6.811	8.465	10.682	21.178	35.187	39.564	43.432
5	10.314	12.377	15.058	26.940	41.639	46.055	49.899
6	14.210	16.636	19.716	32.704	47.807	52.192	55.958
7	18.444	21.191	24.614	38.469	53.735	58.029	61.672
8	22.983	26.011	29.726	44.234	59.449	63.599	67.075
9	27.812	31.083	35.039	50.000	64.961	68.917	72.188
10	32.925	36.401	40.551	55.766	70.274	73.989	77.017
11	38.328	41.971	46.265	61.531	75.386	78.809	81.556
12	44.042	47.808	52.193	67.296	80.284	83.364	85.790
13	50.101	53.945	58.361	73.060	84.942	87.623	89.686
14	56.568	60.436	64.813	78.821	89.318	91.535	93.189
15	63.559	67.381	71.630	84.578	93.333	95.010	96.201
16	71.311	74.988	78.979	90.322	96.827	97.868	98.542
17	80.494	83.843	87.333	96.005	99.382	99.699	99.851

Sample Size = 18

Order Number	2.5	5.0	10.0	50.0	90.0	95.0	97.5
1	0.141	0.285	0.584	3.778	12.008	15.332	18.530
2	1.375	2.011	2.995	9.151	19.947	23.766	27.294
3	3.579	4.702	6.286	14.581	26.942	31.026	34.712
4	6.409	7.970	10.064	20.024	33.441	37.668	41.418
5	9.695	11.643	14.177	25.471	39.602	43.888	47.637
6	13.343	15.634	18.549	30.921	45.502	49.783	53.480
7	17.299	19.895	23.139	36.371	51.184	55.405	59.007
8	21.530	24.396	27.922	41.823	56.672	60.784	64.255
9	26.019	29.120	32.885	47.274	61.980	65.940	69.243
10	30.757	34.060	38.020	52.726	67.115	70.880	73.981
11	35.745	39.216	43.328	58.177	72.078	75.604	78.470
12	40.993	44.595	48.618	63.629	76.861	80.105	82.701
13	46.520	50.217	54.498	69.079	81.451	84.336	86.657
14	52.363	56.112	60.398	74.529	85.823	88.357	90.305
15	58.582	62.332	66.559	79.976	89.936	92.030	93.591
16	65.288	68.974	73.058	85.419	93.714	95.298	96.421
17	72.706	76.234	80.053	90.849	97.005	97.989	98.625
18	81.470	84.668	87.992	96.222	99.416	99.715	99.859

Sample Size = 19

Order Number	2.5	5.0	10.0	50.0	90.0	95.0	97.5
1	0.133	0.270	0.553	3.582	11.413	14.587	17.647
2	1.301	1.903	2.835	8.678	18.977	22.637	26.028
3	3.383	4.446	5.946	13.827	25.651	29.580	33.138
4	6.052	7.529	9.514	18.989	31.859	35.943	39.578
5	9.147	10.991	13.394	24.154	37.753	41.912	45.565
6	12.576	14.747	17.513	29.322	43.405	47.580	51.203
7	16.289	18.750	21.832	34.491	48.856	52.997	56.550
8	20.252	22.972	26.327	39.660	54.132	58.194	61.642
9	24.447	27.395	30.983	44.830	59.246	63.188	66.500
10	28.864	32.009	35.793	50.000	64.207	67.991	71.136
11	33.500	36.812	40.754	55.170	69.017	72.605	75.553
12	38.358	41.806	45.868	60.340	73.673	77.028	79.748
13	43.450	47.003	51.144	65.509	78.168	81.250	83.711
14	48.797	52.420	56.595	70.678	82.487	85.253	87.424
15	54.435	58.088	62.247	75.846	86.606	89.009	90.853
16	60.422	64.057	68.141	81.011	90.486	92.471	93.948
17	66.862	70.420	74.349	86.173	94.054	95.554	96.617
18	73.972	77.363	81.023	91.322	97.165	98.097	98.699
19	82.353	85.413	88.587	96.418	99.447	99.730	99.867

Sample Size = 20

Order Number	2.5	5.0	10.0	50.0	90.0	95.0	97.5
1	0.127	0.256	0.525	3.406	10.875	13.911	16.843
2	1.235	1.807	2.691	8.251	18.096	21.611	24.873
3	3.207	4.217	5.642	13.147	24.477	28.262	31.698
4	5.733	7.135	9.021	18.055	30.419	34.366	37.893
5	8.657	10.408	12.693	22.967	36.066	40.103	43.661
6	11.893	13.955	16.587	27.880	41.489	45.558	49.105
7	15.391	17.731	20.666	32.795	46.727	50.782	54.279
8	19.119	21.707	24.906	37.711	51.803	55.803	59.219
9	23.058	25.865	29.293	42.626	56.733	60.642	63.946
10	27.196	30.195	33.817	47.542	61.525	65.307	68.472
11	31.528	34.693	38.475	52.458	66.183	69.805	72.804
12	36.054	39.358	43.267	57.374	70.707	74.135	76.942
13	40.781	44.197	48.197	62.289	75.094	78.293	80.881
14	45.721	49.218	53.273	67.205	79.334	82.269	84.609
15	50.895	54.442	58.511	72.120	83.413	86.045	88.107
16	56.339	59.897	63.934	77.033	87.307	89.592	91.343
17	62.107	65.634	69.581	81.945	90.979	92.865	94.267
18	68.302	71.738	75.523	86.853	94.358	95.783	96.793
19	75.127	78.389	81.904	91.749	97.309	98.193	98.765
20	83.157	86.089	89.125	96.594	99.475	99.744	99.873

Sample Size = 21

Order Number	2.5	5.0	10.0	50.0	90.0	95.0	97.5
1	0.120	0.244	0.500	3.247	10.385	13.295	16.110
2	1.175	1.719	2.562	7.864	17.294	20.673	23.816
3	3.049	4.010	5.367	12.531	23.405	27.055	30.377
4	5.446	6.781	8.577	17.209	29.102	32.921	36.342
5	8.218	9.884	12.062	21.891	34.522	38.441	41.907
6	11.281	13.245	15.755	26.574	39.733	43.698	47.166
7	14.588	16.818	19.619	31.258	44.771	48.739	52.175
8	18.107	20.575	23.632	35.943	49.661	53.594	56.968
9	21.820	24.499	27.779	40.629	54.416	58.280	61.565
10	25.713	28.580	32.051	45.314	59.046	62.810	65.979
11	29.781	32.811	36.443	50.000	63.557	67.189	70.219
12	34.021	37.190	40.954	54.686	67.949	71.420	74.287
13	38.435	41.720	45.584	59.371	72.221	75.501	78.180
14	43.032	46.406	50.339	64.057	76.368	79.425	81.893
15	47.825	51.261	55.229	68.742	80.381	83.182	85.412
16	52.834	56.302	60.267	73.426	84.245	86.755	88.719
17	58.093	61.559	65.478	78.109	87.938	90.116	91.782
18	63.658	67.079	70.898	82.791	91.423	93.219	94.554
19	69.623	72.945	76.595	87.469	94.633	95.990	96.951
20	76.184	79.327	82.706	92.136	97.438	98.281	98.825
21	83.890	86.705	89.615	96.753	99.500	99.756	99.880

Sample Size = 22

Order Number	2.5	5.0	10.0	50.0	90.0	95.0	97.5
1	0.115	0.233	0.478	3.102	9.937	12.731	15.437
2	1.121	1.640	2.444	7.512	16.559	19.812	22.844
3	2.906	3.822	5.117	11.970	22.422	25.947	29.161
4	5.187	6.460	8.175	16.439	27.894	31.591	34.912
5	7.821	9.411	11.490	20.911	33.104	36.909	40.285
6	10.729	12.603	15.002	25.384	38.117	41.980	45.370
7	13.865	15.994	18.674	29.859	42.970	46.849	50.222
8	17.198	19.556	22.483	34.334	47.684	51.546	54.872
9	20.709	23.272	26.416	38.810	52.275	56.087	59.342
10	24.386	27.131	30.463	43.286	56.752	60.484	63.645
11	28.221	31.126	34.619	47.762	61.119	64.746	67.790
12	32.210	35.254	38.881	52.238	65.381	68.874	71.779
13	36.355	39.516	43.248	56.714	69.537	72.869	75.614
14	40.658	43.913	47.725	61.190	73.584	76.728	79.291
15	45.128	48.454	52.316	65.666	77.517	80.444	82.802
16	49.778	53.151	57.030	70.141	81.326	84.006	86.135
17	54.630	58.020	61.883	74.616	84.998	87.397	89.271
18	59.715	63.091	66.896	79.089	88.510	90.589	92.179
19	65.088	68.409	72.106	83.561	91.825	93.540	94.813
20	70.839	74.053	77.578	88.030	94.883	96.178	97.094
21	77.156	80.188	83.441	92.488	97.556	98.360	98.879
22	84.563	87.269	90.063	96.898	99.522	99.767	99.885

Sample Size = 23

Order Number	2.5	5.0	10.0	50.0	90.0	95.0	97.5
1	0.110	0.223	0.457	2.969	9.526	12.212	14.819
2	1.071	1.567	2.337	7.191	15.884	19.020	21.949
3	2.775	3.652	4.890	11.458	21.519	24.925	28.038
4	4.951	6.168	7.808	15.734	26.781	30.364	33.589
5	7.460	8.981	10.971	20.015	31.797	35.493	38.781
6	10.229	12.021	14.318	24.297	36.626	40.390	43.703
7	13.210	15.248	17.816	28.580	41.305	45.098	48.405
8	16.376	18.634	21.442	32.863	45.856	49.644	52.919
9	19.708	22.164	25.182	37.147	50.291	54.046	57.226
10	23.191	25.824	29.027	41.431	54.622	58.315	61.458
11	26.820	29.609	32.971	45.716	58.853	62.461	65.505
12	30.588	33.515	37.012	50.000	62.988	66.485	69.412
13	34.495	37.539	41.147	54.284	67.029	70.391	73.180
14	38.542	41.685	45.378	58.569	70.973	74.176	76.809
15	42.734	45.954	49.709	62.853	74.818	77.836	80.292
16	47.081	50.356	54.144	67.137	78.558	81.366	83.624
17·	51.595	54.902	58.695	71.420	82.184	84.752	86.790
18	56.297	59.610	63.374	75.703	85.682	87.979	89.771
19	61.219	64.507	68.203	79.985	89.029	91.019	92.540
20	66.411	69.636	73.219	84.266	92.192	93.832	95.049
21	71.962	75.075	78.481	88.542	95.110	96.348	97.225
22	78.051	80.980	84.116	92.809	97.663	98.433	98.929
23	85.151	87.788	90.474	97.031	99.543	99.777	99.890

Sample Size = 24

Order Number	2.5	5.0	10.0	50.0	90.0	95.0	97.5
1	0.105	0.213	0.438	2.847	9.148	11.735	14.247
2	1.026	1.501	2.238	6.895	15.262	18.289	21.120
3	2.656	3.495	4.682	10.987	20.685	23.980	26.997
4	4.735	5.901	7.473	15.088	25.754	29.227	32.361
5	7.132	8.589	10.497	19.192	30.588	34.181	37.384
6	9.773	11.491	13.694	23.299	35.246	38.914	42.151
7	12.615	14.569	17.033	27.406	39.763	43.469	46.711
8	15.630	17.796	20.493	31.513	44.160	47.873	51.095
9	18.799	21.157	24.058	35.621	48.449	52.142	55.322
10	22.110	24.639	27.721	39.729	52.641	56.289	59.406
11	25.553	28.236	31.476	43.837	56.742	60.321	63.357
12	29.124	31.942	35.317	47.946	60.755	64.244	67.179
13	32.821	35.756	39.245	52.054	64.683	68.058	70.876
14	36.643	39.679	43.258	56.163	68.524	71.764	74.447
15	40.594	43.711	47.359	60.271	72.279	75.361	77.890
16	44.678	47.858	51.551	64.379	75.942	78.843	81.201
17	48.905	52.127	55.840	68.487	79.507	82.204	84.370
18	53.289	56.531	60.237	72.594	82.967	85.431	87.385
19	57.849	61.086	64.754	76.701	86.306	88.509	90.227
20	62.616	65.819	69.412	80.808	89.503	91.411	92.868
21	67.639	70.773	74.246	84.912	92.527	94.099	95.265
22	73.003	76.020	79.315	89.013	95.318	96.505	97.344
23	78.880	81.711	84.738	93.105	97.762	98.499	98.974
24	85.753	88.265	90.852	97.153	99.562	99.787	99.895

Sample Size = 25

Order Number	2.5	5.0	10.0	50.0	90.0	95.0	97.5
1	0.101	0.205	0.421	2.735	8.799	11.293	13.719
2	0.984	1.440	2.148	6.623	14.687	17.612	20.352
3	2.547	3.352	4.491	10.553	19.914	23.104	26.031
4	4.538	5.656	7.166	14.492	24.802	28.172	31.219
5	6.831	8.229	10.062	18.435	29.467	32.961	36.083
6	9.356	11.006	13.123	22.379	33.966	37.541	40.704
7	12.072	13.948	16.317	26.324	38.331	41.952	45.129
8	14.950	17.030	19.624	30.270	42.582	46.221	49.388
9	17.972	20.238	23.032	34.215	46.734	50.364	53.500
10	21.125	23.559	26.529	38.161	50.795	54.393	57.479
11	24.402	26.985	30.111	42.108	54.722	58.316	61.335
12	27.797	30.513	33.774	46.054	58.668	62.138	65.072
13	31.306	34.139	37.514	50.000	62.486	65.861	68.694
14	34.928	37.862	41.332	53.946	66.226	69.487	72.203
15	38.665	41.684	45.228	57.892	69.889	73.015	75.598
16	42.521	45.607	49.205	61.839	73.471	76.441	78.875
17	46.500	49.636	53.266	65.785	76.968	79.762	82.028
18	50.612	53.779	57.418	69.730	80.376	82.970	85.050
19	54.871	58.048	61.669	73.676	83.683	86.052	87.928
20	59.296	62.459	66.034	77.621	86.877	88.994	90.644
21	63.917	67.039	70.533	81.565	89.938	91.771	93.169
22	68.781	71.828	75.198	85.508	92.834	94.344	95.462
23	73.969	76.896	80.086	89.447	95.509	96.648	97.453
24	79.648	82.388	85.313	93.377	97.852	98.560	99.016
25	86.281	88.707	92.201	97.265	99.579	99.795	99.899

Appendix 3

Standards and Regulatory Organization Addresses

Note: Telephone numbers are listed using the ISO standard method showing: Country Code + Area/City Code + Number.

American National Standards Institute (ANSI)
1430 Broadway
New York, NY 10018, USA
Ph: +1+212+354-3300

American Society for Quality Control (ASQC)
310 W. Wisconsin Avenue
Milwaukee, WI 53203, USA
Ph: +1+414+272-8575

American Society for Testing Materials (ASTM)
1916 Race Street
Philadelphia, PA 19103, USA
Ph: +1+215+299-5400

Association for the Advancement of Medical Instrumentation (AAMI)
3330 Washington Boulevard, Suite 400
Arlington, VA 22201-4598, USA
Ph: +1+703+525-4890

Association Francaise de Normalisation Tour Europe (AFNOR)
Tour Europe, La Defense
F-92080 Paris, France
Ph: +33+1+4291-5555

British Standards Institute (BSI)
2 Park Street
London W1A 2BS, United Kingdom
Ph: +44+71+629-9000

Canadian Standards Institute (CSI)
178 Rexdale Boulevard
Rexdale, ON, M9W 1R3 Canada
Ph: +1+416+747-4379

Comitato Electrotecnico Italiano
20126 Milano
Vialle Mon Za, 00259, Italy
Ph: +39+2+575-841

Department of Health (DOH)
14 Russell Square
London WC1B 5EP United Kingdom
Ph: +44+1+636-6811

Deutsches Institut fur Normung (DIN)
Postfach 1107
D-1000 Berlin 30, West Germany
Ph: +49+30+2601-1

European Committee for Electrotechnical Standardization (CENELEC)
2 Rue de Brederode
B-1000 Brussels, Belgium
Ph: +32+2+511-7932

European Committee for Standardization (CEN)
2 Rue de Brederode
B-1000 Brussels, Belgium

Food and Drug Administration (FDA)
5600 Fishers Lane
Rockville, MD 20857, USA
Ph: +1+301+443-1544

Institute of Electrical and Electronic Engineers (IEEE)
345 East 47th Street
New York, NY 10017, USA
Ph: +1+212+705-7908

Instituto Espanol de Normalization (AENOR)
Fernandez del la Hoz, 52
E-28010 Madrid, Spain
Ph: +34+1+410-4851

Instrument Society of America (ISA)
67 Alexander Drive
P.O. Box 12277 Research Triangle Park, NC 27709, USA
Ph: +1+919+549-8411

International Electrotechnical Commission (IEC)
3 Rue de Varembe
CH-1211 Geneva 20, Switzerland
Ph: +41+22+734-0150

International Organization for Standardization (ISO)
1 Rue de Varembe
CH-1211 Geneva 20, Switzerland
Ph: +41+22+343-1240

International Special Committee on Radio Interference
3 Rue de Varembe
CH-1211 Geneva 20, Switzerland
Ph: +41+22+734-1240

Japanese Standards Association (JSA)
1-24 Akasaka 4, Minato-ku
Tokyo 107, Japan
Ph: +81+3+583-8001

Joint Commission on Accredidation of Healthcare Organizations
875 N. Michigan Avenue
Chicago, IL 60611, USA
Ph: +1+312+642-6061

National Electrical Manufacturers Association (NEMA)
2101 L Street NW
Washington, DC 20037, USA
Ph: +1+202+457-8473

National Fire Protection Association (NFPA)
Batterymarch Park
Quincy, MA, 02269, USA
Ph: +1+800+344-3555

Standards Association of Australia (SAA)
P. O. Box 458
North Sydney, NSW 2059, Australia
Ph: +61+2+963-4111

Suomen Standardisoimisliitto (SFS)
P.O. Box 205
SF-00121 Helsinki 12, Finland
Ph: +358-0-645-601

Swedish Planning and Rationalization Institute for the
  Health and Social Services
Box 27310
S-102 54 Stockholm, Sweden

Underwriters Laboratory (UL)
1285 Walt Whitman Road
Melville, NY 11747, USA
Ph: +1+516+271-6200

Verband Deutscher Elektrotechniker (DKE)
Stresemannallee 15
D-6000 Frankfurt am Main 70, West Germany
Ph: +49+69+63080

Appendix 4

Reliability Glossary

ACCELERATED TESTING:
Testing at a higher than normal stress level to increase the failure rate and shorten the time to wearout.

ACCEPTABLE RELIABILITY LEVEL (ARL):
A nominal failure rate specified for the acceptance of parts or equipment.

ACCESSIBILITY:
A measure of the relative ease of admission to the various areas of an item for the purpose of operation or maintenance.

AMBIENT:
Used to denote surrounding, encompassing or local conditions and is usually applied to enviroments, e.g., ambient temperature, ambient pressure.

ARITHMETIC MEAN:
The sum of a set of values divided by the number in the set.

AVAILABLE TIME:
The period that elapses from completion of corrective action or preventative maintenance to the next critical failure or preventative maintenance action.

AVERAGE:
A value which represents or summarizes some relevant feature of a set of values. Sometimes used for arithmetic mean.

BREADBOARD MODEL:
An assembly in rough form to prove the feasibility of a circuit, device, system or principle.

BURN-IN:
The operation of an item to stabilize its characteristics.

CALENDAR AGE:
Age measured in terms of time since the object was manufactured.

CATASTROPHIC FAILURE:
A sudden change in the operating characteristic of an item resulting in a complete lack of useful performance of the item.

CHANCE FAILURE:
Any failure which is not induced by external phenomena.

CHARACTERISTIC:
Any dimensional, visual, functional, mechanical, electrical, chemical, physical or material feature or property. Any process-control element which describes and establishes the design, fabrication and operation of an article.

CHECKOUT:
Tests or observations of an item to determine its condition or status.

CHECKOUT TIME:
Time required to determine whether the performance characteristics of a system are within specified values.

COMPLEXITY:
The figure of merit or measure of the quantity of related parts or circuits.

COMPONENT FAILURE:
A failure of any component to perform one or more of its design functions satisfactorily when subjected to an enviroment within its design limitations.

COMPUTED RELIABILITY:
The calculated probability of a system or a device with a system performing its purpose within specifications based on estimates or tests of the reliability of its parts.

CONDITIONING:
The exposure of sample units or specimens to a specific enviroment for a specified period of time to prepare them for subsequent inspection.

CONFIDENCE:
The probability that may be attached to conclusions reached as a result of application of statistical techniques.

CONFIDENCE INTERVAL:
The numerical range within which an unknown is estimated to be.

CONFIDENCE LEVEL:
The probability that a given statement is correct. The probability that a stated confidence interval includes an unknown.

CONFIDENCE LIMITS:
The extremes of a confidence interval within which the unknown has a designated probability of being included.

CONFIGURATION:
A listing of the assemblies which comprise a device.

CONSTANT FAILURE RATE:
A failure rate which is invariant during a period of a device's life.

CONTINUOUS VARIABLE:
A variable that may assume any value within a defined range.

CONTROLLED TEST:
A sampling method designed to solve a problem or group of problems concerning a given product.

CORRECTIVE ACTION:
A documented design, process, procedure or materials change implemented and validated to correct the cause of failure or design deficiency.

CORRECTIVE MAINTENANCE:
That maintenance performed on a nonscheduled basis to restore equipment to satisfactory conditions.

CORRELATION:
A relationship between two variables.

CREEP
Continuous increase in deformation under constant or decreasing stress. The term is ordinarily used with reference to the behavior of metals under tension at elevated temperatures.

For plastic material, an initial strain proportional to the modulus of elasticity, followed by a slow but steady increase in strain with time. The combination of plastic flow and elastic deformation expressed as the sum of the initial strain plus the incremental strain which occurs with time at constant stress.

CRITICAL ITEM:
An item whose failure could result in hazardous or unsafe conditions or prevent performance of the basic function of the end item.

CYCLE:
An ON/OFF application of power. A change in state and back again.

DAMAGE:
A degree of physical harm to an item which, without repair, renders it unsuitable for its intended use.

DEBUGGING:
A process to detect and remedy inadequacies.

DEFECT:
Any imperfection, fault, flaw, lack of completeness or other conditions at variance with technical requirements.

DEFICIENCY:
A general term covering any defect, failure, discrepancy or other lack of conformance to specifications.

DEGRADATION:
A gradual deterioration in performance.

DEGRADATION FACTOR:
A factor by which reliability of an item is reduced in processing, handling, usage, etc.

DEGRADATION FAILURE:
A failure that results from a gradual change in performance characteristics with time.

DEMONSTRATED:
That which has been measured by the use of objective evidence gathered under specified conditions.

DERATING:
Using an item in such a way that applied stresses are below rated values.

The lowering of the rating of an item in one stress field to allow an increase in another stress field.

DESIGN EVALUATION:
An evaluation to determine whether the design of a product meets the design criteria established as necessary to provide a product which will meet the needs of the user.

DESTRUCTIVE TESTING:
Testing of any sort which drastically degrades the item tested.

DEVIATION:
An approved departure from specification requirements.

DEVICE:
Any functional system.

DISCRETE VARIABLE:
A variable which can take only a finite number of values.

DOWN TIME:
The total time during which the system is not in condition to perform its intended function.

DURABILITY:
A measure of useful life.

DUTY CYCLE:
A specified operating time of an equipment plus a specified time of nonoperation.

EARLY FAILURE PERIOD:
An interval immediately following final assembly, during which the failure rate of certain items is relatively high.
A synonym for the infant mortality period.

ENVIRONMENT:
The aggregate of all conditions which externally influence the performance of an item.

FAIL-SAFE:
The stated condition that the equipment will contain self- checking features which will cause a function to cease in case of failure, malfunction or drifting out of tolerance.

FAILURE:
An event or inoperable state, in which any item or part of an item does not, or would not, perform as previously specified.

FAILURE ANALYSIS:
Subsequent to a failure, the logical systematic examination of any item, its construction, application and documentation to identify the failure mode and determine the failure mechanism.

FAILURE, CATASTROPHIC:
A failure that can cause item loss.

FAILURE DATA:
A collection of discrepancy and malfunction data derived from test and field experiences.

FAILURE, INTERMITTENT:
Failure for a limited period of time, followed by the item's recovery of its ability to perform within specified limits without any remedial action.

FAILURE MECHANISM:
The physical, chemical, electrical, thermal or other process which results in failure.

FAILURE MODE:
The consequence of the mechanism through which the failure occurs.

FAILURE RATE:
The probability of failure per unit of time of the items still operating.

FATIGUE:
A weakening or deterioration of metal or other material, or of a member, occurring under load, especially under repeated, cyclic or continued loading.

FAULT:
Immediate cause of failure.

FAULT ISOLATION:
The process of determining the location of a fault to the extent necessary to effect repair.

FEASIBILITY STUDY:
The study of a proposed item or technique to determine the degree to which it is practicable, advisable and adaptable for the intended purpose.

INHERENT FAILURE:
A failure basically caused by a physical condition or phenomenon internal to the failed item.

INHERENT RELIABILITY:
Reliability potential present in the design.

INHERENT SAFETY:
Safety features that automatically arise from the design of a device.

MAINTAINABILITY:
The measure of the ability of an itme to be retained in or restored to specified condition when maintnenace is performed by personnel having specified skill levels, using prescribed procedures and resources, at each prescribed level of maintenance and repair.

MAINTENANCE:
The servicing, repair and care of material or equipment to sustain or restore acceptable operating conditions.

The repair, reconstruction and care required to keep an installation in operating condtion.

MAINTENANCE, CORRECTIVE:
All actions performed as a result of failure to restore an item to a specified condition. Corrective maintenance can include any or all of the following steps: localization, isolation, disassembly, interchange, reassembly, alignment and checkout.

MAINTENANCE, PREVENTATIVE:
All actions performed in an attempt to retain an item in specified condition by providing systematic inspection, detection and prevention of incipient failures.

MAINTENANCE, SCHEDULED:
Preventive maintenance performed at prescribed points in the item's life.

MALFUNCTION:
Any occurrence of unsatisfactory performance.

MANUFACTURABILITY:
The measure of the design's ability to consistently satisfy product goals, such as technical performance, quality, reliability availability and cost, while being profitable.

MEAN:
Usually refers to an arithmetic mean.

MEAN TIME BETWEEN FAILURE (MTBF):
A basic measure of reliability for repairable items.

The mean number of life units during which all parts of the item perform within their specified limits during a particular measurement interval, under stated conditions.

MEAN TIME BETWEEN MAINTENANCE (MTBM):
A measure of the reliability taking into account maintenance policy. The total number of life units expended by a given time, divided by the total number of maintenance events due to that item.

MEAN TIME TO FAILURE (MTTF):
A basic measure of maintainability.

The sum of repair times divided by the total number of failures, during a particular interval under stated conditions.

MEAN TIME TO REPAIR (MTTR):
The sum of repair times divided by the total number of failures, during a particular interval under stated conditions.

MEDIAN:
The middle value of a set of values.

MINIMUM LIFE:
The time of occurrence of the first failure of a device.

MODE:
The unit of a set of values which occurs most often.

MODULE:
A replaceable combination of assemblies, subassemblies and parts common to one mounting.

NON-DESTRUCTIVE TESTING:
Testing of any nature which does not materially affect the life expectancy of the item tested.

NULL HYPOTHESIS:
A negative proposition used for the purpose of a statistical test.

OPERABLE:
The state of being able to perform the intended function.

OPERATING TIME:
> The time period between turn-on and turnoff of a system, sub-system, component or part during which time operation is as specified.

PARAMETER:
> A quantity to which the operator may assign arbitrary values, as distinguished from a variable, which can assume only those values that the form of the function makes possible.

PART FAILURE:
> A failure which usually involves a non-repairable breakdown and immediate end of life for a part which is subsequently permanently replaced.

PERFORMANCE STANDARDS:
> Published instructions and requirements setting forth the procedures, methods and techniques for measuring the designed performance of equipments or systems in terms of the main number of essential technical measurements required for a specified operational capacity.

POPULATION:
> The total collection of units being considered.

PRECISION:
> The degree to which repeated observations of a class of measurements conform to themselves.

PREDICTED:
> That which is expected at some future time, postulated on analysis of past experience and tests.

PROBABILITY:
> A measure of the likelihood of any particular event occurring.

PROBABILITY DISTRIBUTION:
> A mathematical model which represents the probabilities for all of the possible values a given discrete random variable may take.

PROTOTYPE:
> A model suitable for use in complete evaluation of form, design and performance.

QUALIFICATION:
> Formal assurance and approval that an article used in the device meets all operational and reliability requirements under all conditions of expected environment.

QUALITY:
  a. The extent to which a device conforms to specifications.

  b. The proportion of satisfactory devices in a lot.

REDUNDANCY:
  Duplication, or the use of more than one means of performing a function in order to prevent an overall failure in the event that all but one of the means fails.

REDUNDANCY, ACTIVE:
  That redundancy wherein all redundant items are operating simultaneously.

REDUNDANCY, STANDBY:
  That redundancy wherein the alternative means of performing the function is not operating until it is activated upon failure of the primary means of performing the function.

REGRESSION ANALYSIS:
  The fitting of a curve or equation to data in order to define the functional relationship between two or more correlated variables.

RELIABILITY:
  The probability that a device will perform a required function, under specified conditions, for a specified period of time.

RELIABILITY DESIGN REVIEW:
  An evaluation of a system and/or its components for the purpose of recommending design changes which will improve reliability. The evaluation gives due consideration to other design criteria, including producibility, schedules, cost, weight, size, performance and maintainability.

RELIABILITY GOAL:
  The desired reliability for the device.

RELIABILITY GROWTH:
  The improvement a reliability parameter caused by the successful correction of deficiencies in item design or manufacture.

RELIABILITY TEST:
  Tests designed to measure the level and uniformity of reliability.

REPAIR:
  All actions performed as a result of failure, to restore an item to a specified condition.

RISK:
The probability of making an incorrect decision.

SAFETY FACTOR:
The margin of safety designed into theapplication of an item to insure that it will function properly.

SAMPLE:
A set of product specimen chosen to represent all units in a batch.

SAMPLE SIZE:
The number of sample units in a sample.

SCREENING:
A process of inspecting items to remove those that are unsatisfactory or those likely to exhibit early failure.

SERVICEABILITY:
Requirements to be met by equipment design, configuration, installation and operation that will minimize maintenance requirements.

SERVICING:
The performance of any act needed to keep an item in operating condition, but not including preventative maintenance of parts or corrective maintenance tasks.

SERVICE LIFE:
The design operating life time of the equipment, beyond the occurrence of which continued maintenance and logistic support becomes economically unjustifiable.

SHELF LIFE:
The length of time an item can be stored under specified conditions and still meet specified requirements.

SIMULATION:
A set of test conditions designed to duplicate field operating and usage environments as closely as possible.

SINGLE POINT FAILURE:
The failure of an item which would result in failure of the system and is not compensated for by redundancy or alternative operational procedures.

SPECIFICATION:
A detailed description of the characteristics of a product and of the criteria which must be used to determine whether the product is in conformity with the description.

STANDARD DEVIATION:
A statistical measure of dispersion in a distribution.

STATISTICS:
The science of collection, presentation, analysis and interpretation of numerical data.

SYSTEM:
A system is a group of equipments, including any required operator functions, which are integrated to perform a related operation.

SYSTEM COMPATIBILITY:
The ability of the equipments within a system to work together to perform the intended mission of the system.

TOLERANCE:
The allowable variations in measurements within which an item is judged acceptable.

TRADE-OFF:
The lessening of some desirable factor(s) in exchange for an increase in one or more other factors to maximize a system's effectiveness.

VARIABLE:
A quantity that may assume a number of values.

VARIANCE:
A statistical measure of the dispersion in a distribution.

WEAROUT:
The process which results in an increase of the failure rate or probability of failure with increasing number of life units.

WEAROUT FAILURE PERIOD:
The period of equipment life following the normal failure period, during which the equipment failure rate increases above the normal rate.

WORST CASE CIRCUIT ANALYSIS:
A type of circuit analysis that determines the worst possible effect on the output parameters by changes in the values of circuit elements. The circuit elements are set at the values within their anticipated ranges which produce the maximum detrimental output changes.

Index

Accelerated testing, 131
Acceptance testing, 152
Active redundancy, 61
Antistatic control, 196
Application stresses, 72
Applied load, 72
Assembly, 193
Association for the Advancement of Medical Instrumentation, 30
Audit evaluation, 199
Beta contract, 163
Beta evaluation, 163
Black box testing, 149
Block diagram, 61
Bottom up design, 100
Bovie units, 162
British Standards Institute, 30
Burn-in activity, 191
Canadian Standards Association, 29
Catastrophic failures, 16
Chance or random failures, 16
Change control procedures, 199
Chi-square table, 117, 223
Class I medical devices, 25
Class I recalls, 216
Class II medical devices, 26
Class II recalls, 216
Class III medical devices, 26

Class III recalls, 216
Coding, 109
Combined loads, 73
Complaint handling, 199, 213
Component activity, 190
Component classification, 70
Component derating, 71
Component failure rate, 69, 77
Component history, 69
Component qualification, 191
Component reliability, 67
Component safety, 69
Component selection, 64
Component testing, 151
Computer aided metrics, 107
Conditional release, 189
Conducted emissions, 162
Conducted susceptibility, 162
Confidence level, 117, 176
Confidence limits, 177
Cooper Committee, 25
Cost, 96
Critical component, 65
Critical device, 66
Criticality, 65
Curved plots, 138, 182
Customer service, 46
Customer survey, 49
Cycle testing, 121

Data analysis, 169, 205
Defect, 14
Deficiency, 14
Definition of reliability, 4
Degradation failure, 17
Design, 43, 55, 59, 93
Design errors, 108
Design review, 56, 86, 101
Device Reconditioner/Rebuilder
  (DRR), 26
Device history record, 214
Device reliability, 9
Drift failure, 17
Dynamic burn-in, 192
Early failures, 7, 15
Electromagnetic compatibility,
  161
Electronic reliability, 6
Electrostatic discharge, 74, 161,
  195
Environmental conditions, 74
Environmental testing, 115,
  156
European Committee for
  Electrotechnical
  Standardization, 32
European Community, 33
European Free Trade Area, 38
Event testing, 115
Failure, 15
Failure analysis, 46, 195, 211
Failure definition, 15, 116, 150
Failure investigation, 215
Failure investigation and
  analysis system, 199
Failure mode analysis, 70, 151
Failure modes and effects
  analysis, 70, 128, 212
Failure rate, 19, 169
Failure related testing, 115
Failure terminated, 172, 173

Failure terminated confidence
  limits, 178
Fault, 14
Fault tree analysis, 69, 103, 122
FDA, 1, 23, 65, 96, 196
FDA Form 483, 200
Feasibility, 43, 49
Federal Food, Drug and
  Cosmetic Act (FFD&C), 24
Feedback, 46, 219
Field failure analysis, 212
Field operation, 46, 203
Field service reports, 203
Final release, 189
Fitness for use, 64
510(k), 44
Food and Drug Administration
  (FDA), 1, 23, 65, 96, 196
Freedom of Information Act, 200
Frequency sweep, 159
GIDEP (Government-Industry
  Data Exchange Program), 69
Glossary, 245
GMP inspections, 198
Good Manufacturing Practices
  (GMP), 26, 46, 196
Graphical analysis, 179
Graphical plots, 209, 213
Graphical plotting, 181
Ground mobile, 77
Halstead measures, 106
Hard failure, 150
Hardware validation, 44, 113
Hardware/software compatibility,
  55, 155
Health Industry Manufacturers
  Association (HIMA), 98
History of reliability, 2
Humidity, 74
Humidity testing, 157
ISO 9000, 36

Impact testing, 160
Incoming requirements, 190
Increasing sample size, 131
Increasing test severity, 131
Infant mortality, 7, 10, 15
Initial vendor assessment, 67
Institute of Electrical and
  Electronic Engineers, 32
Integration testing, 151
Intermittent failure, 17
International Electrotechnical
  Commission, 28
International Organization for
  Standardization, 32
International Special Committee
  on Radio Interference, 31
Japanese Engineering Standards
  Committee, 33
Japanese Industrial Standards
  Committee, 33
Japanese Standards Association,
  33
Kiviat diagrams, 107
Length of burn-in, 192
Length of the program, 106
Liability cases, 95
Linear plots, 138, 182
Load protection, 73
Location parameter, 134, 182
Logic symbols, 123
Long term reliability testing,
  114
Lot control, 191
Malfunction, 14
Manufacturing, 45, 187
McCabe's Complexity, 105
Mean Time Between Failure
  (MTBF), 20, 52, 62, 77, 84,
  116, 121, 135, 165, 170, 182
Mechanical impact, 74, 160
Mechanical reliability, 8

Mechanical shock, 74
Mechanical shock testing, 159
Mechanical vibration, 74
Mechanical vibration testing,
  134
Median rank, 141
Medical device, 25
Medical Device Amendments to
  the FFD&C Act, 1, 25
Medical Device Reporting
  (MDR), 26, 214
MIL-HDBK-217, 20, 44, 62, 69,
  75, 124
Minimum life, 179
Modes of failures, 123
Module interaction, 100
National Electronic
  Manufacturers Association
  (NEMA), 98
National Fire Protection
  Association, 29
Omission of symbols, 108
Operating temperature, 75
Operating temperature testing,
  156
Operational failures, 16
Operational stress level, 72
Operational stresses, 72
Overstress testing, 115
Packaged vibration, 159
Pareto analysis, 179, 209
Pareto charts, 212
Parts count prediction, 77
Percent rank tables, 225
Plot, 182, 209, 213
Population line, 144
Potential hazards, 103
Premarket approval, 44
Preventive maintenance, 46
Product development cycle, 41
Product development process, 41

Product life cycle, 42, 219
Product misuse, 74
Product recalls, 215
Product release, 187
Product release review, 187
Product Specification, 43, 50, 55 116
Product validation, 45, 155
Project team, 41, 187
Quality, 3
Quality assurance, 198
Radiated emissions, 162
Radiated susceptibility, 162
Random vibration, 159
Real time logic, 103, 104
Recalls, 199
Record Retention Policy, 200
Redundancy, 61
Reliability, 4, 20, 84, 175
Reliability assurance, 5
Reliability calculations, 152, 175
Reliability demonstration, 165
Reliability goal, 51
Reliability optimization, 10
Reliability plan, 56
Reliability report, 57
Repair, 21
Resonant frequencies, 160
Revision level control, 193
Risk assessment, 61
Risk level, 176
Safety, 59, 95
Safety analysis, 162
Safety margin, 72
Sample size, 116
Sanctions, 200
Scale parameter, 134, 182
Serious injury, 214
Shape parameter, 134, 138, 182
Single point failure, 128
Soft failure, 150

Software, 93, 147, 193
Software Quality Assurance, 98, 108
Software failures, 108, 150
Software metrics, 104
Software policy, 96
Software reliability, 9, 93
Software reviews, 101
Software safety, 103
Software specification, 99, 193
Software validation, 44, 147
Software verification, 147
Specification errors, 108
Specification review, 53, 56, 101
Standard tests, 121
Standards and regulatory organization addresses, 241
Standby redundancy, 63
Static burn-in, 192
Statistical Process Control (SPC), 46, 195
Storage temperature, 74
Storage temperature testing, 157
Structured approach, 100
Structured manufacturing process, 189
Structured software testing, 151
Sudden death band lines, 144
Sudden death line, 141
Sudden death testing, 133, 138
System, 103
System burn-in, 194
System specification, 43, 55
System testing, 151
10 × 10 testing, 121
Test and inspection, 193
Test completion criteria, 149
Test fixtures, 193
Test protocol, 114, 119
Test time, 116
Thermal shock testing, 157

Time Petri net models, 104
Time Petri nets, 103
Time related testing, 115
Time terminated, 171, 172
Time terminated confidence
  limits, 177
Top down design, 100
Track I inspections, 198
Track II inspections, 198
Trend analysis, 199
Trending, 211, 215
Type of test, 114
Types of burn-in, 192
Typical use testing, 121
Typographical errors, 108
Underwriters Laboratory, 28
Unreliability, 3
Useful life, 7, 10, 16, 134
Validation, 44
Validation phase, 113, 147, 155,
  169
Validation protocol, 114, 148, 193

Validation software review, 153
Validation testing, 113
Vendor audit, 67
Vendor evaluation, 67
Vendor qualification, 67
Verification, and validation plan,
  148
Verification and validation
  report, 152
Vocabulary of the software,
  106
Volume of software, 107
Warranty analysis, 213
Warranty cost, 52, 84, 211
Wearout, 7, 10, 16
Wearout failures, 16
Weibull analysis, 134, 182
Weibull distribution, 134, 182
Weibull plotting, 134, 182
White box testing, 149
Written procedures, 197